RAPID INTERPRETATION

OF

EKG's

. . . a programmed course

By

Dale Dubin, M.D.

All illustrations and graphic art were produced by the author.

Published by:
COVER Publishing Company
P.O. Box 1092
TAMPA, FLORIDA 33601
U.S.A.

Telephones
In U.S. 1-800-441-8398
Outside U.S. 813-237-0266
FAX 813-238-1819

ALL FOREIGN LANGUAGE EDITIONS GRANTED BY EXCLUSIVE IMPRIMATUR
OF COVER PUBLISHING CO., COVER INC., USA

Library of Congress Catalog Card Number 88-072108
ISBN 0-912912-01-4

Cover Publishing International Distribution

The English edition of *Rapid Interpretation of EKG's* can be purchased through any of our worldwide distribution/fulfillment centers:

Central America

Casa Medica
Guatemala

South America

Carlos Hirsch SRL
Buenos Aires, Argentina

Libreria Uniandes
Bogota, Columbia

BECO Internacional
LaPaz, Bolivia

COLIVRO
Rio de Janeiro, Brazil

Australia/New Zealand

University Co-Op Bookshop
Broadway, N.S.W., Australia

Bennett's Bookshop
Palmerston North, New Zealand

Norfold Bookstore
Lower Hutt, New Zealand

Indonesia

Schmidt Scientific Sdn. Bhd.
Kuala Lumpur, Malaysia

Southeast Asia

Asia Books Co. Ltd.
Bangkok, Thailand

Orient

M & Vactek Corp.
Taipei, Taiwan

Japan

Yohan Western Dist. Agency
Tokyo, Japan

Soviet Union

Mezhdunarodnaya Kniga
Moscow, U.S.S.R.

Eastern Europe

Slovart Co. Ltd.
Bratislava, Czechoslovakia

Ars Polona
Warsaw, Poland

United States/Canada

Cover Publishing Company
Tampa, FL   33601, USA

Middle East

Atha Electronics
Athens, Greece

Garmac Medical Equipment
Haifa, Israel

Sifri/Yakir
Tel-Aviv, Israel

World of Knowledge
Jeddah, Saudi Arabia

United Kingdom

H. K. Lewis and Company
London, England

University Bookshop
Belfast, Northern Ireland

Europe

ACCO Boekhandel
Leuven, Belgium

Kunst und Wissen
Stuttgart, West Germany

Scandinavia

Vingmed Svenska AB
Jarfalla, Sweden

Turun Kansallinen Kirjakauppa
Turku, Finland

Akateeminen Kirjakauppa
Helsinki, Finland

Iceland

Boksala Studenta
Reykjavik, Iceland

Austurbakki hf.
Reykjavik, Iceland

Africa

P. B. Mayer Books
Cape Town, South Africa

P. J. DeVilliers Bookshop
Bloemfontein, South Africa

Westdene-Rondebosch Bookshop
Rondebosch, South Africa

Literary Group
Braammfontein, South Africa

. . . and with profound gratitude to those who took personal time to scrutinize and provide tracings of pathology; they (absent degrees and titles) are herein acknowledged for their altruism which should be appreciated through the ages:

M. Schloss, New York University Medical Center, New York, NY.; Columbia Hospital, Milwaukee, WI.; S. Schulz, Mount Carmel Mercy, Detroit, MI.; L. Berrien, Cottage Hospital, Santa Barbara, CA.; L. Shannon, The Medical Center, Beaver, PA.; L. Mulloy, El Camino Hospital, Mount View, CA.; L. Cosgrove, Winthrop University Hospital, Mineola, Long Island, NY.; P. Rosier, Berkshire Medical Center, Pittsfield, MA.; L. S. DeWitt, Daniel Freeman Memorial Hospital, Inglewood, CA.; G. Larrivee, University of Massachusetts Medical Center, Worcester, MA.; University of California San Diego Medical Center, San Diego, CA.; Valley Hospital, Ridgewood, NJ.; M. Puskar, Veterans Administration Hospital, Pittsburgh, PA.; D. M. Glover, Saint Francis Medical Center, Trenton, NJ.; R. W. Fugate, Richmond, VA.; K. L. Briggs, LaCross, WI.; P. A. Mullen, Nazareth Hospital, Philadelphia, PA.; F. Ward, Jr., Methodist Hospital, Lubbock, TX.; M. A. Gildea, Rogue Valley Medical Center, Medford, OR.; C. J. Todd, Methodist Hospital, Indianapolis, IN.; E. Amicucci, Saint Vincent Health Center, Erie, PA.; D. Novak, Oak Park Hospital, Oak Park, IL.; J. Frost, University of California San Diego, San Diego, CA.; St. Joseph's Hospital of Atlanta, Atlanta, GA.; RHM, Columbia, SC.; G. Galucci, Brooklyn, NY.; S. Ciccotto, VA Medical Center, Northport, NY.; S. Walker, Oklahoma City, OK.; M. Brennan, Daniel Freeman Hospital, Inglewood, CA.; East Jefferson General Hospital, Metairie, LA.; S. Brandley, Providence Medical Center, Seattle, WA.; J. Kushner, LDS Hospital, Salt Lake City, UT.; C. Katanski, VA Medical Center, Allen Park, MI.; Schumpert Medical Center, Shreveport, LA.; Battle Mountain General Hospital, Battle Mountain, NV.; C. Gazgano, Montefiore Medical Center, Bronx, NY.; R. L. O'Bryant, Menorah Medical Center, Kansas City, MO.; J. A. Dimeo, St. Francis Health System, Pittsburgh, PA.; Abbott Northwestern Hospital, Minneapolis, MN.; Jefferson Hospital, Pittsburgh, PA.; F. Kim and S. B. Cope, St. Louis, MO.; T. Hill, Sinai Hospital of Detroit, Detroit, MI.; N. Slone, Wadsworth, IL.; B. Elash, Tucson Medical Center, Tucson, AZ.; C. Ferenczy, University of California Irvine, Orange, CA.; P. L. Brown, Olin Teague Veterans Center, Temple, TX.; B. Helms, Fayette, AL.; D. K. DeArment, Altoona Hospital, Altoona, PA.; D. Buechi-Burton, San Diego, CA.; D. L. Ohlrogge, St. Lukes Hospital, Denver, CO.; N. Davis, Inglewood, CA.; Doctors Hospital, Little Rock, AR.; K. Thompson, Medical City Dallas, Dallas, TX.; B. Koehler, Harrison, OH.; D. Anderson, North Colorado Medical Center, Greeley, CO.; E. Reker, Allentown Hospital, Allentown, PA.; E. M. Elinson, Woburn, MA.; C. Hartigan, St. Elizabeth's Hospital of Boston, Brighton, MA.; L. Brown, VA Hospital, Indianapolis, IN.; D. Bergman, St. Paul Medical Center, Forney, TX.; The Lower Bucks Hospital, Bristol, PA.; R. M. Scott, Wake Medical Center, Raleigh, NC.; K. Hojnowski and D. Ellis, Virginia Commonwealth University, Richmond, VA.; S. Parr, St. Francis Medical Center, Peoria, IL.; J. Dwyer, Deaconess Hospital, Evansville, IN.; Mississippi Baptist Medical Center, Jackson, MS.; H. Reese, Geisinger Medical Center, Danville, PA.; S. E. Furedy, Phoenix, AZ.; VA Medical Center, Allen Park, MI.; B. Mammen, Clayton General Hospital, Riverdale, GA.; N. Miller, York Hospital, York, PA.; C. Bohnet, Flint Osteopathic Hospital, Flint, MI.; L. Salmon, Brackenridge Hospital, Austin, TX.; VA Medical Center, Allen Park, MI.; St. Lukes Regional Medical Center, Sioux City, IA.; C. Pate, Medical College of Georgia, Augusta, GA.; M. Mahoney, K. Gage, M. Cerruda, Rhode Island Hospital, Providence, R.I.; Barbara Caldbech, St. Lukes Hospital, Cedar Rapids, IA.; Cheryl Daniel, Jasper, FL.; Mary Gelliarth, Tampa General Hospital, Tampa, FL.; Cary D. Snow, ZMI Corporation, Cambridge, MA.; J. Wines, Marquette Electronics Inc., Milwaukee, WI.

ACKNOWLEDGMENTS

With humility and gratitude I acknowledge my indebtedness:

To God for the inspiration, to fate for the expiration.

To all my mentors from whom I have learned principles of electrocardiography.

To Martha and Sam for their perseverance and longevity.

To Samantha and Amanda for their indefatigable faith.

To my publisher, COVER Publishing Company, for their great understanding and cooperation. My association with the publisher represents the closest possible concert between author and publisher.

DEDICATION

To Those From Whom I Have Learned:

Dr. Paul Dudley White
Dr. George C. Griffith
Dr. Willard J. Zinn
Dr. Henry J. L. Marriott
Dr. Charles Fisch
Dr. William L. Martz
Dr. Nathan Marcus
Dr. Richard G. Connar
Dr. Jose Dominguez
Dr. Louis Cimino
Dr. David Baumann
Dr. Suzanne Knoeble
Dr. Dale Dubin

TABLE OF CONTENTS

"To make a great dream come true, the first requirement is a great capacity to dream; the second is persistence—a faith in the dream."

Hans Selye, M.D.

Before You Begin . . .

First read each caption and associate it with the graphic illustration.

    Master each illustration.

Then carefully read the programmed text, filling in each blank as you go.

- If you have to return to the illustration to refresh your memory—that's even better—. . . because each time you review an illustration, the visual image will be more indelibly impressed in your memory.
- Programmed instruction is intellectual growth by graduated increments of related concepts.

    . . . and it works because it is really an exciting audience participation course, and you are the audience.

"Lasting knowledge results from understanding."

Happy Learning,

Dale Dubin, M.D.

Most teachers are knowledgable.
Good teachers are intelligent.
Great teachers are patient.
Exceptional teachers are students themselves.
        D.D.

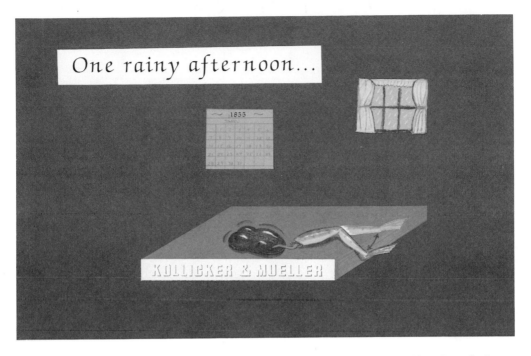

One rainy afternoon...

1855

KOLLICKER & MUELLER

While dissecting live frogs, around 1855, Kollicker and Mueller found that when a motor nerve to a frog's leg was laid over the isolated beating heart, the leg kicked with each heartbeat.

Eureka! they thought, the same electrical stimuli which
cause the leg to kick, must cause the _____ to beat.   heart

> NOTE: By the way, it was already known that an
> electrical stimulus applied to a motor nerve causes
> contraction of the associated muscle (thanks to the work of
> Luigi Galvani a century before).

So it was logical for them to assume that the beating
of the heart must be due to a rhythmic discharge of
_____ stimuli . . .   electrical

. . . and that's how basic research begins.*

*Wouldn't a warm cup of coffee be nice right now?

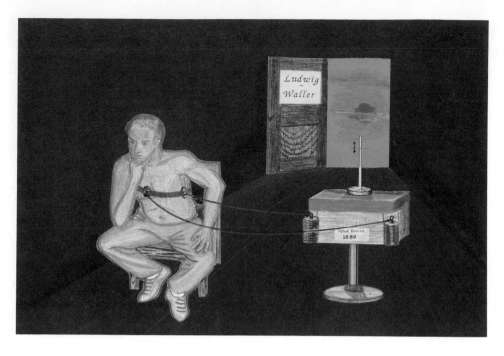

In the mid 1880's Ludwig and Waller found that the heart's rhythmic electrical stimuli could be monitored from a person's skin.

Their basic device had sensor electrodes which were placed on a man's _____ and connected to a capillary tube in an electrical field.

skin

The level of fluid in the capillary tube moved with the rhythm of the subject's _____-beat . . . very interesting.

heart

They called this device the "capillary electrometer" and it was a little too unsophisticated for clinical application or even for economic exploitation, but it *was* _____ interesting.

very

NOTE: And most of all, it opened the door for monitoring the electrical activity of the heart from (intact) skin surfaces.

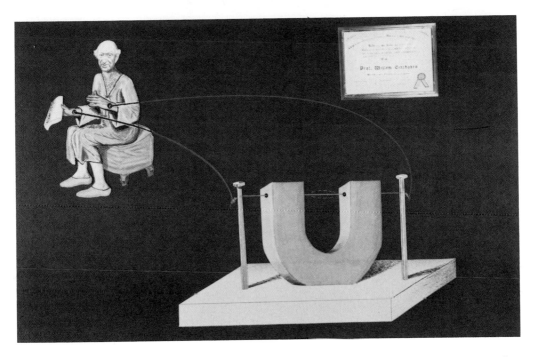

Enter Einthoven, a brilliant man who took a large permanent magnet and suspended a silvered wire through holes drilled in both poles of the magnet.

Two skin sensors (electrodes) placed on a man were then connected across the silvered wire which ran between two poles of the _____.   magnet

The silvered _____ (suspended in the magnetic field)   wire danced rhythmically to the subject's heartbeat.

This was also very interesting, but _____   Einthoven wanted a timed record of these events. So . . .

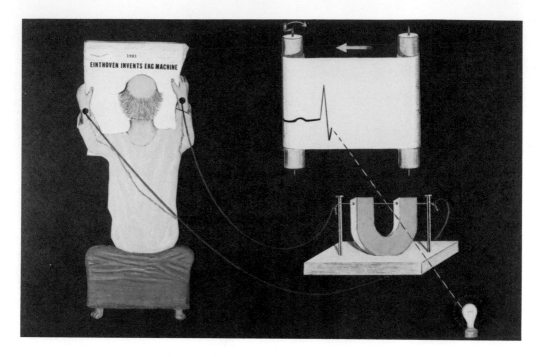

So Einthoven projected a tiny light beam across the dancing silvered wire, and its rhythmic movements were recorded as waves on a scroll of moving photographic paper.

Very clever that Einthoven! The _____ rhythmic
movements of the wire (representing the heartbeat) created
a bouncing shadow.

. . . which was recorded as a _____ series of rhythmic
distinct waves in repeating cycles.

The _____ of each cardiac cycle were named waves
(alphabetically) P, QRS, and T.

> NOTE: "Now," thought the clever Einthoven, "we can
> record the heart's *abnormal* electrical activity—and
> compare it with the normal." And so a great diagnostic
> tool, the "electro**k**ardiogram," evolved around 1901. Let's
> see how it works . . .

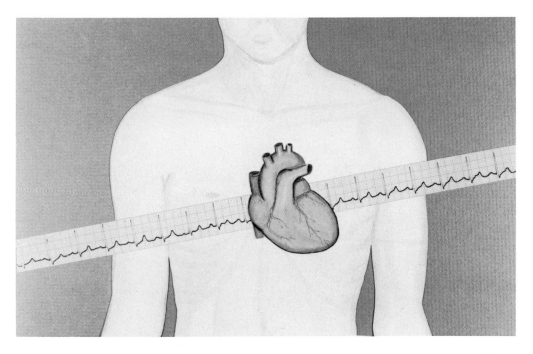

The electrocardiogram (EKG) records the electrical activity of the heart, providing a valuable, permanent record of its function.

The electrocardiogram is commonly known by the three letters _____, and gives us valuable information concerning the heart's function.

EKG

NOTE: Since the time of Einthoven, the medical profession has used the letters EKG to represent electrocardiogram. The "K" replacing the "C" of "cardio" avoids confusion with EEG (brain wave recording) because ECG and EEG sound alike. Some purists claim ECG is more correct, but we will continue to refer to the electrocardiogram as an EKG since this term has been used extensively for many years, and Medicine honors tradition.

The electrocardiogram is inscribed on a ruled paper strip and gives us a permanent _____ of cardiac activity. Cardiac monitors display the same activity.

record

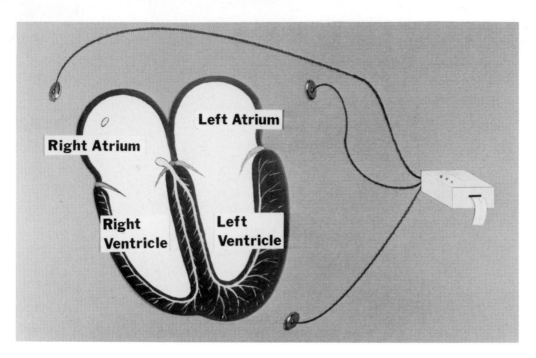

The electrocardiogram records the electrical impulses that stimulate the heart to contract.

The information recorded on the EKG represents the
_____ impulses from the heart.   electrical

Most of the electrical impulses represent various stages of
cardiac _____.   stimulation

>   NOTE: The EKG also yields valuable information on the
>   heart during resting and recovery phases.

When the heart muscle is electrically stimulated, it
_____.   contracts

>   NOTE: The main purpose of this illustration is to
>   familiarize you with the diagramatic cross section of the
>   heart which will be used continuously throughout this
>   book. You probably could have recognized the various
>   chambers without the labels, but I added them anyway.

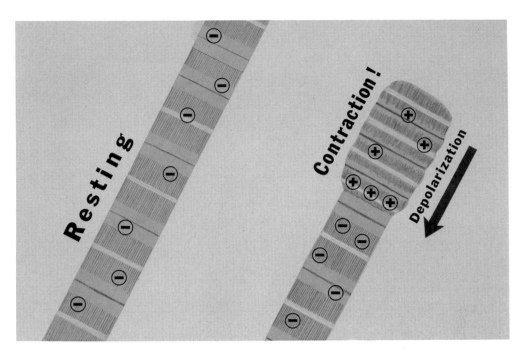

Muscle cells of the heart are charged or polarized in the resting state, but when they depolarize, this electrical stimulus causes their contraction.

In the resting state the cells* of the heart are polarized, the inside of the cells being _____ charged.

negatively

> NOTE: In the strictest sense, a resting, polarized cell has a negatively charged interior and a positively charged surface. For the sake of simplicity we will consider only the inside of the myocardial cell.

The interiors of the myocardial cells, which are usually negatively charged, become _____-ly charged as the cells are stimulated to contract.

positive

The electrical stimulation of the heart's muscle cells is called "depolarization" and causes them to _____.

contract

*The muscle cells of the heart are often referred to as "myocardial" cells, and collectively they are called the myocardium.

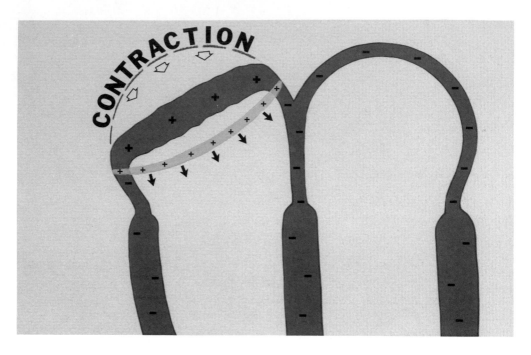

Thus a progressive wave of stimulation (depolarization) passes through the heart causing contraction of the myocardium.

This depolarization may be considered an advancing wave of _____ charges within the cells.

positive

NOTE: Depolarization stimulates the myocardial cells to contract as the charge within each cell changes to positive.

The electrical stimulus of depolarization causes progressive contraction of the _____ cells as the wave of positive charges advances down the interior of the cells.

myocardial

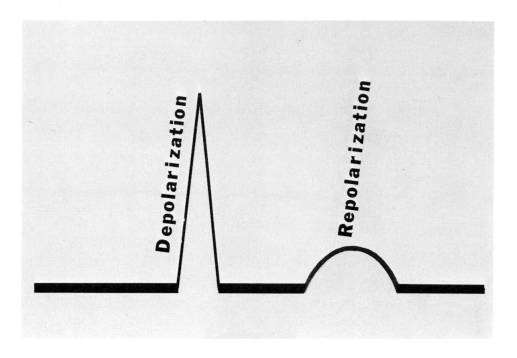

The wave of depolarization (cells become positive inside), and the phase of repolarization (cells return to negative) which follows, are recorded on the EKG as shown.

The stimulating wave of depolarization charges the interior of the myocardial cells _____-ly and stimulates them to contract.

positive

But during the phase of _____, the myocardial cells regain the negative charge within each cell.

repolarization

NOTE: Repolarization is a strictly electrical phenomenon, the myocardial cells do not respond to repolarization.

Myocardial stimulation, or _____, and the recovery phase, or _____, are recorded on the EKG as shown.

depolarization
repolarization

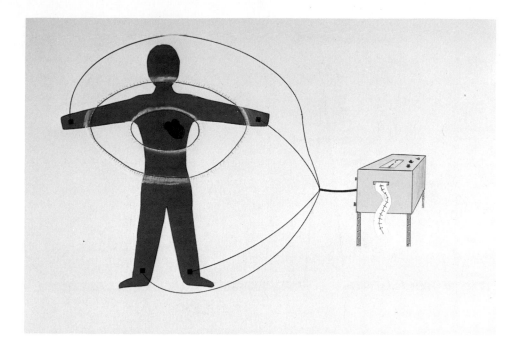

As this electrical activity passes through the heart, it can be detected by external (skin) sensors and recorded as an EKG.

NOTE: These skin sensors are often called "electrodes."

Both depolarization and repolarization are
_____ phenomena.   electrical

The electrical activity of the heart may be detected and
recorded from the _____ surface by sensitive monitoring   skin
equipment.

The EKG records the electrical activity of the heart from
electrode _____ placed on the skin.   sensors

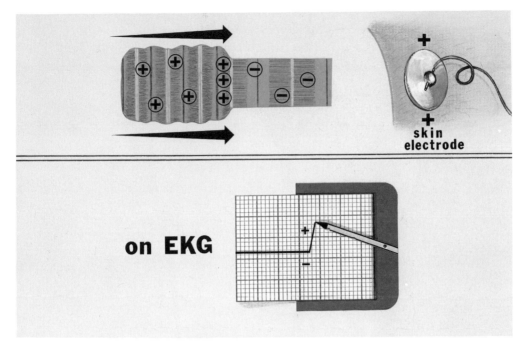

As the positive wave of depolarization within the heart cells moves toward a positive (skin) electrode, there is a positive (upward) deflection recorded on EKG.

An advancing wave of depolarization may be considered a moving wave of _____ charges.   positive

When this wave of positive charges is moving toward a positive _____ electrode, there is a simultaneous upward deflection recorded on EKG.   skin

When there is a depolarization stimulus moving toward a positive skin electrode, a _____ (upward) wave is recorded on the electrocardiogram.   positive

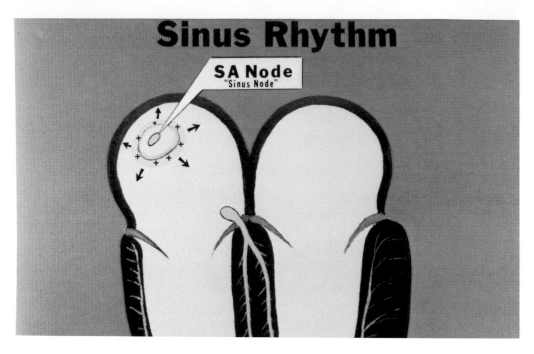

The *SA Node* begins the electrical impulse which spreads outward in wave fashion, stimulating both atria to contract.

NOTE: The SA Node ("Sinus Node") is the heart's natural pacemaker, so its pacing activity is known as a "Sinus Rhythm".

The SA Node, located within the upper-posterior wall of the right _____, initiates the electrical impulse for cardiac stimulation.

atrium

This wave of depolarization proceeds outward from the SA Node and stimulates both _____ to contract.

atria

As this depolarization wave passes through the atria, it produces a concurrent wave of atrial

_____.

contraction

NOTE: The electrical stimulus originating in the SA Node proceeds away from the Node in all directions. If the atria were a pool of water and a pebble dropped at the SA Node, an enlarging circular wave would spread out from the SA Node. This is the manner in which atrial depolarization proceeds away from the SA Node. Remember that atrial depolarzation is a spreading wave of positive charges within the myocardial cells.

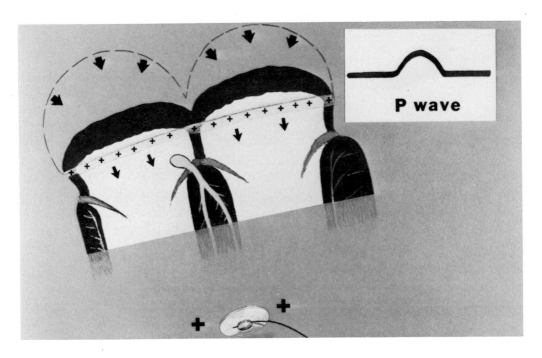

This electrical impulse spreads through the atria and yields a *P wave* on the EKG.

The wave of depolarization sweeping through the _____ can be picked up by the sensitive skin sensors.

atria

This atrial stimulation is recorded as a ____ wave on EKG.

P

The P wave represents atrial _____ electrically.

depolarization
(stimulation)

NOTE: The illustration depicts the positive wave of atrial depolarization advancing toward a positive electrode, producing an upward (positive) P wave on EKG.

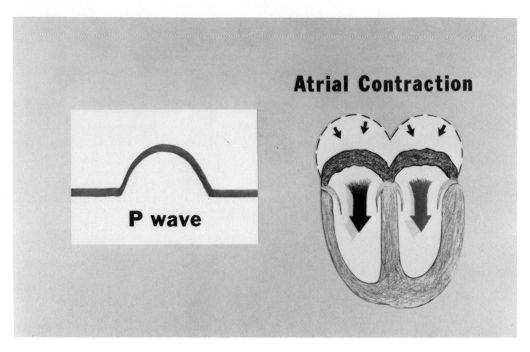

Thus the P wave represents the electrical activity of the contraction of both atria.

As the wave of depolarization passes through both atria, there is a simultaneous wave of atrial

_____.   contraction

So the P wave represents the depolarization and contraction of both _____.   atria

> NOTE: In reality contraction lags slightly behind depolarization, but we will consider both to be occurring simultaneously.

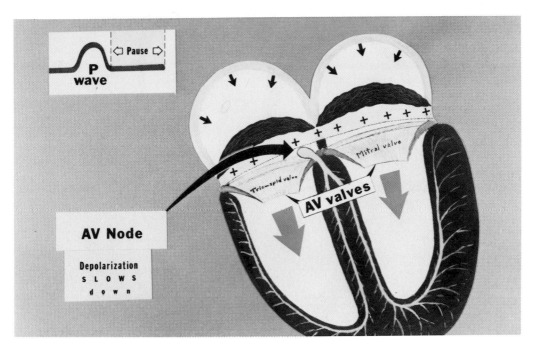

The impulse then reaches the *AV Node* where there is a brief pause, allowing blood to enter the ventricles.

This stimulating wave of depolarization eventually reaches the _____, the only electrical pathway between the atria and the ventricles.

AV Node

Once the AV Node is stimulated, there is a _____ before the impulse of depolarization can completely penetrate through the AV Node (because the stimulus of *depolarization slows within the AV Node*).

pause

This brief pause allows the blood from the atria to pass through the AV valves* into the _____.

ventricles

NOTE: At this point we are correlating these electrical phenomena with the mechanical physiology. The atria contract forcing blood through the AV valves, but it takes a little time for the blood to travel through the valves into the ventricles (thus the pause which produces the short piece of flat baseline after each P wave).

*There is a (one-way) AV valve between each atrium and its associated ventricle. These valves allow the blood to pass only from the atria to the ventricles, therefore backflow is prevented.

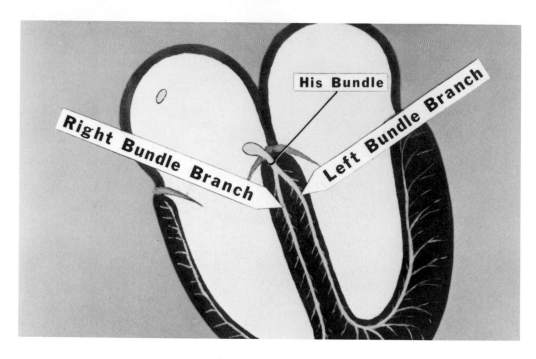

Although depolarization slows within the AV Node, this stimulus of depolarization proceeds rapidly down the *His Bundle* into the *Bundle Branches*.

Although the stimulus is retarded in passage through the AV Node, this depolarization stimulus continues through the _____ _____ rapidly.

His Bundle

This electrical stimulus passes slowly through the AV Node, then rapidly down the His Bundle to the Left and Right _____ Branches.

Bundle

After the stimulus has rapidly progressed through the His Bundle and the Bundle Branches, depolarization can be distributed to the myocardial cells of the _____.

ventricles

NOTE: The His Bundle (bundle of His), which extends down from the AV Node, divides into Right and Left Bundle Branches within the interventricular septum.

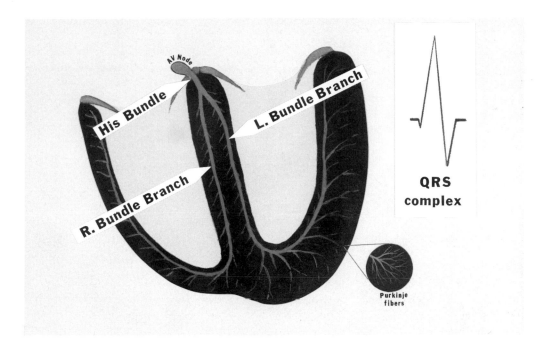

The electrical stimulus is distributed via the terminal *Purkinje fibers* to the ventricular myocardial cells, and it is the depolarization of the myocardial cells which produces a *QRS complex* on EKG tracing.

NOTE: The *ventricular conduction system* is composed of specialized nervous tissue which rapidly carries the electrical impulse (depolarization) away from the AV Node. The ventricular conduction system consists of the His Bundle, and the Right and Left Bundle Branches terminating in the fine Purkinje fibers. Depolarization moves much more rapidly through this specialized nervous tissue than is possible through the myocardial cells alone. The [rapid] passage of the stimulus down the ventricular conduction system does *not* record on EKG.

Once an electrical impulse emerges from the AV Node, it progresses rapidly through the His Bundle to the Right and Left Bundle Branches into the _____ fibers which terminate in the ventricular myocardial cells.

Purkinje

The QRS complex represents ONLY the depolarization of the myocardial _____ of the ventricles.

cells

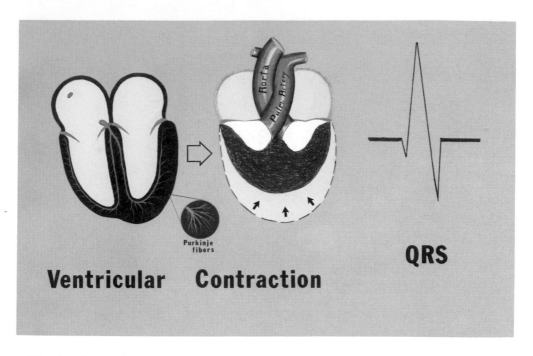

The Purkinje fibers transmit the electrical impulse (depolarization) to the myocardial cells, causing ventricular contraction, and producing a QRS complex on the tracing.

The fine Purkinje fibers transmit this _____ electrical
stimulus directly to the myocardial cells.   (or depolarization)

Thus the impulse transmitted to the ventricular myocardial
cells causes contraction of the _____ and   ventricles
produces a QRS complex on the tracing.

> NOTE: The QRS complex on an EKG represents the
> beginning of ventricular contraction. The physical act of
> ventricular contraction actually lasts longer than the QRS
> complex, but we will consider the QRS complex to
> represent ventricular contraction. So the QRS complex
> represents depolarization of the ventricules, which causes
> ventricular contraction. Still with me?

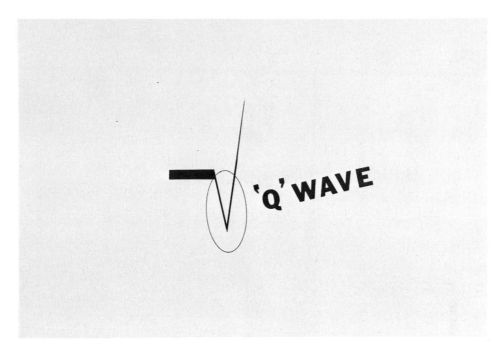

The *Q wave* is the first downward stroke of the QRS complex, and it is followed by the upward *R wave*. The Q wave is often not present.

The Q wave is a wave which moves _____ on the tracing.   downward

The Q wave, when present, occurs at the _____ of the QRS complex and is the first   beginning
downward deflection of the complex.

The downward Q wave is followed by an upward _____   R
wave.

> NOTE: If there is any upward deflection in a QRS complex that appears before a "Q" wave, it is not a Q wave, for by the definition the Q wave is the first wave of the QRS complex. The Q wave is always the first wave in the complex when it is present.

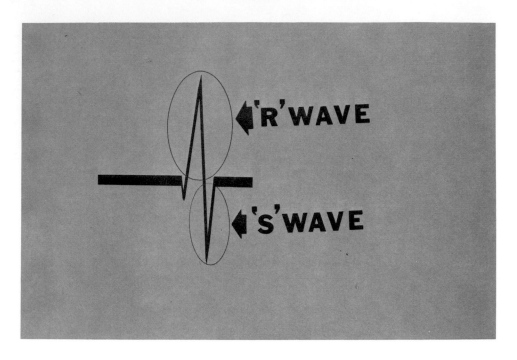

The upward R wave is followed by a downward *S wave*. This total QRS complex represents the electrical activity of ventricular depolarization.

The first upward deflection of the QRS complex is the
_____ _____.

R wave

Any downward stroke *PRECEDED* by an upward stroke is an _____ _____.

S wave

The complete QRS complex can be said to represent _____ depolarization (and the initiation of ventricular contraction).

ventricular

> NOTE: The upward deflection is always called an R wave. Distinguishing the downward Q and S waves really depends on whether the downward wave occurs before or after the R wave. The Q occurs before the R wave and the S wave is after the R.

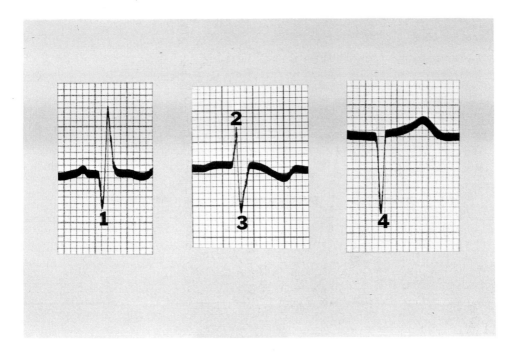

Name each of the above numbered waves.

1. _____.   Q

2. _____.   R

3. _____.   S

4. _____.   QS

NOTE: Number 4 was a little unfair. Because there is no
upward wave, we cannot determine whether number 4 is a
Q wave or an S. Therefore it is called, appropriately, a *QS
wave* and is considered to be a Q wave when we look for
Q's.

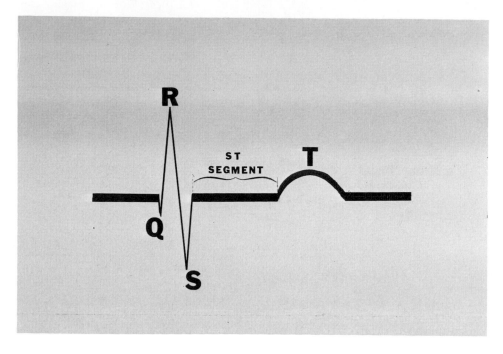

There is a pause after the QRS complex, then a *T wave* appears.

There is a _____ after the QRS complex.   pause

This pause is the ____ _____.   ST segment

> NOTE: This *ST segment*, which is merely the flat piece of
> baseline between the QRS complex and the T wave, is
> pretty darn important as you will soon see.

So after the QRS complex there is a (usually flat) ST
segment which is followed by the ____ wave.   T

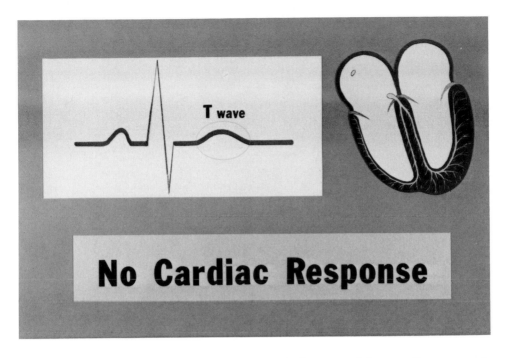

T wave

No Cardiac Response

The T wave represents repolarization of the ventricles so they may be stimulated again.

The T wave represents ventricular
_____.   repolarization

Repolarization occurs so that the myocardial cells can
regain the negative charge within each _____, so they   cell
can be depolarized again.

> NOTE: The ventricles have no physical response to
> repolarization. This is strictly an electrical phenomenon
> recorded on EKG. The atria also have a repolarization
> wave which is very small and usually lost within the QRS
> complex and therefore not seen ordinarily.

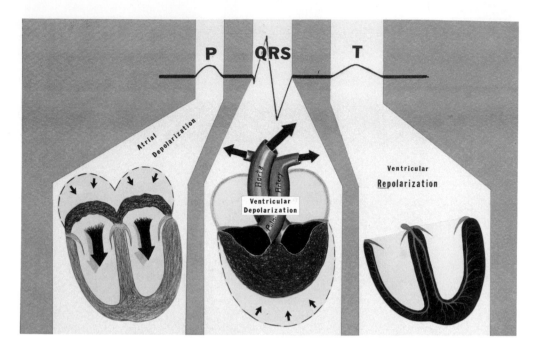

One cardiac cycle is represented by the P wave, QRS complex, and T wave. This cycle is repeated continuously.

Atrial depolarization and contraction is represented by the _____ wave.

P

Ventricular depolarization and contraction is represented by the _____ _____.

QRS complex

NOTE: Physiologically a cardiac cycle represents atrial systole (atrial contraction), ventricular systole (ventricular contraction), and the resting stage that follows.

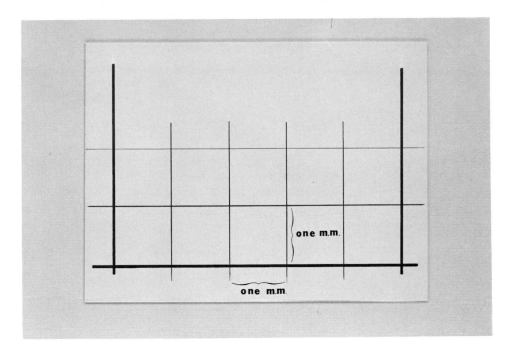

The EKG is recorded on ruled (graph) paper. The smallest divisions are one millimeter squares.

The electrocardiogram is recorded on a long strip of
_____ paper.   ruled (or graph)

The smallest divisions are _____ _____   one millimeter
long and _____ _____ high.   one millimeter

There are _____ small squares between the heavy   five
black lines.

> NOTE: This strip of graph paper moves leftward under the recording needle, and similarly on cardiac monitor the display moves leftward.

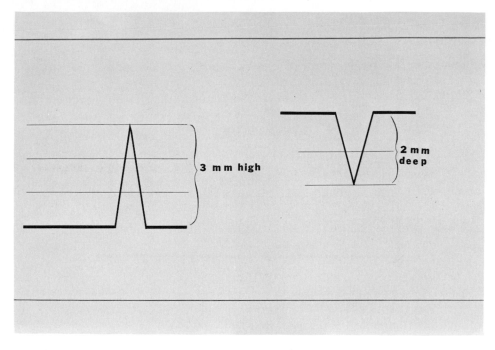

The height and depth of a wave are measured in millimeters and this represents a measure of voltage.

The height or depth of waves may be measured in
_____.   millimeters

The height and depth of waves measure the
_____.   voltage

The elevation or depression of segments of baseline is
similarly _____ in millimeters* just as we   measured
measure waves.

*Millimeters is abbreviated mm.

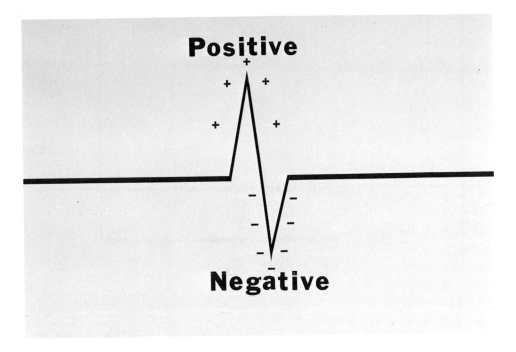

Upward deflections are called "positive" deflections. Downward deflections are called "negative" deflections on EKG's.

Positive deflections are _____ on the EKG.   upward

Negative deflections are _____ on the EKG.   downward

NOTE: When a wave of stimulation (depolarization) advances toward a positive skin sensor (electrode), this produces a positive (upward) deflection on EKG. You will recall that depolarization is an advancing wave of positive charge within the cells. So with depolarization the advancing wave of positive charge creates a positive deflection on EKG when this wave is moving toward a positive skin sensor. Be Positive! (If you're still a little shaky on this point return to page 11 momentarily.)

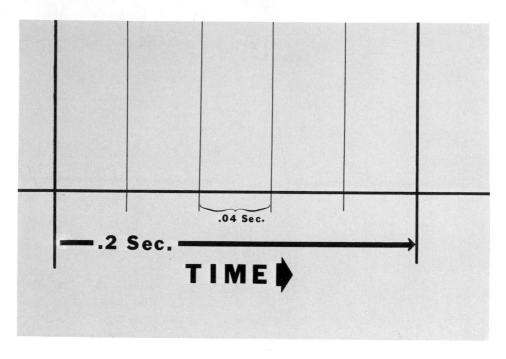

The horizontal axis represents time.

The amount of time represented by the distance between
the heavy black* lines is _____.

.2 of a second
(2/10 of a second)

There are _____ small squares between the heavy black
lines.

five

Each small division (when measured horizontally between
the fine lines) represents _____.

.04 of a second
(that's 4
hundredths!)

*EKG paper is now printed in a variety of colors, so the heavy lines may not be black.

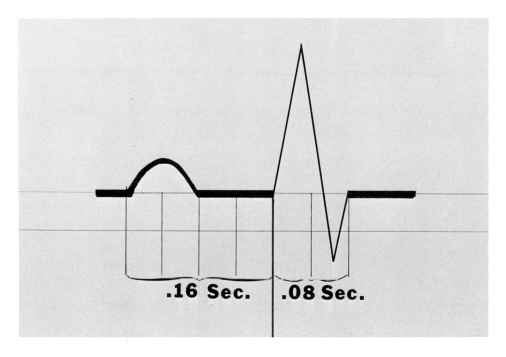

By measuring along the horizontal axis, we find the duration of any part of the cardiac cycle.

The duration of any wave may be determined by measuring along the horizontal _____.

axis

Four of the small squares represent _____ second.

.16
(16 hundredths)

The amount of graph paper which passes under a point in .12 second is _____ small squares. (You don't have to be a mathematician to read EKG's.)

three

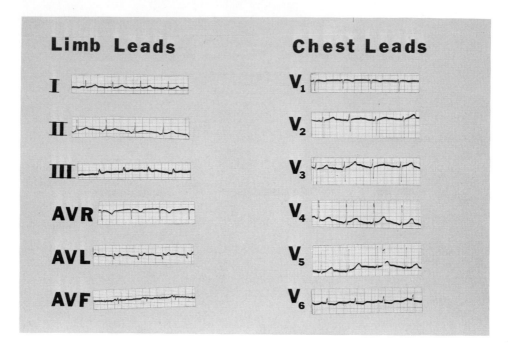

The standard EKG is composed of 12 separate *leads**.

The standard EKG is composed of six _____ leads
and six _____ leads.

chest
limb

> NOTE: Leads not considered "standard" can be monitored
> from various locations on the body.

*Rhymes with seeds.

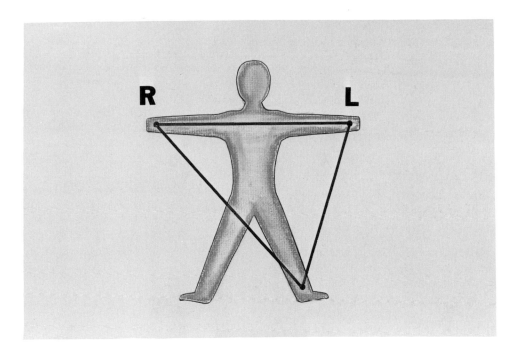

To obtain the *limb leads*, electrodes are placed on the right and left arms and the left leg forming a triangle (Einthoven's)*.

By placing electrodes on the right and left arms and the left leg, we can obtain the _____ leads.   limb

The placement of these electrodes forms a
_____.   triangle

NOTE: The electrocardiogram was historically monitored by using these three locations for the electrode sensors.

*After Dr. Willem Einthoven who invented the EKG machine in 1901.

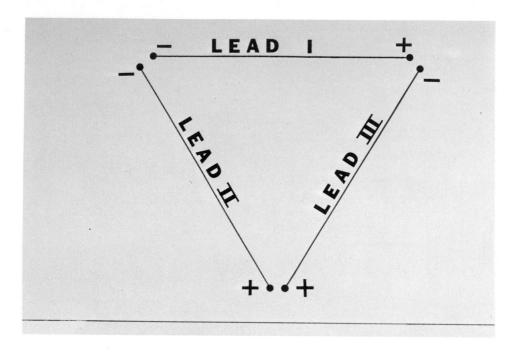

Each side of the triangle is formed by two electrodes and represents a limb lead. By using a different pair of electrodes for each lead, this makes three separate limb leads (lead I, lead II, and lead III) for monitoring.

A pair of electrodes forms a limb _____.   lead

These leads consist of a pair of electrodes, one is always
positive, and one is _____, so they are   negative
sometimes called "bipolar" limb leads.

Lead I is horizontal and the left arm sensor is
_____ while the right arm sensor is   positive
_____.   negative

> NOTE: The engineering wonders of the EKG machine
> permit us to make any skin sensor positive or negative
> depending on which pair of electrodes (i.e., lead) the
> machine is monitoring.*

When we consider lead III, the left arm sensor is now
_____ and the left leg sensor is   negative
_____.   positive

*In reality, an electrode sensor is placed on the right leg as well for EKG monitoring. This helps
stabilize the tracing.

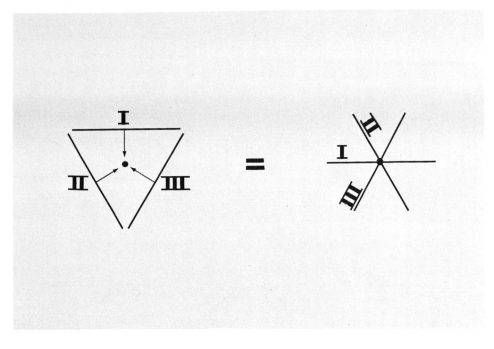

By pushing these three limb leads to the center of the triangle, we have three intersecting lines of reference.

The triangle has a center and each _____ may be moved to that center point.

lead

By pushing limb leads I, II, and III to the center of the triangle, three intersecting lines of _____ are formed.

reference

Although the leads are moved to the _____ of the triangle, they remain at the same angle. (It's still the same leads yielding the same information.)

center

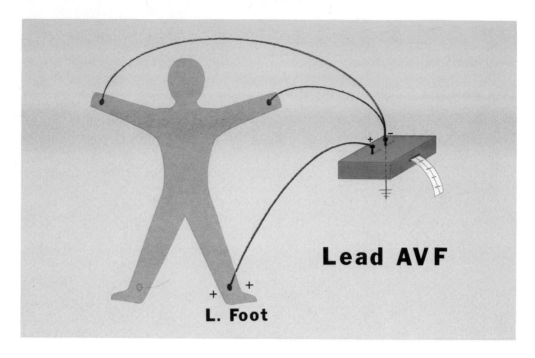

Lead AVF

L. Foot

Another lead is the AVF lead. The AVF lead uses the left Foot as positive and *both* arm electrodes as a common ground (negative). Lets forget the right foot for now.

The AVF lead uses the left Foot as _____.   positive

The right arm and left arm _____ are   sensors
channeled into a common (negative) ground.   (electrodes)

> NOTE: Dr. E. Goldberger who introduced the "Augmented"
> limb leads, discovered that in order to monitor a lead in
> this manner he had to amplify (Augment) the Voltage in
> the EKG machine to get a tracing of the same magnitude
> as leads I, II, and III. He named the lead A (<u>A</u>ugmented),
> V (<u>V</u>oltage), F (left <u>F</u>oot), and he also created two more
> leads using the same technique.

> ASIDE: Your deductive mind will tell you that lead AVF
>   is a mixture of leads II and III . . . just what Dr.
>   Goldberger was trying to accomplish. Therefore
>   lead AVF is a cross between (and oriented
>   between) those two bipolar leads. Now let's create
>   two more Augmented leads.

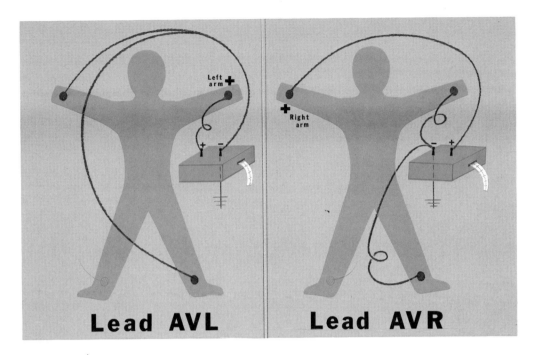

Lead AVL   Lead AVR

The remaining two augmented limb leads, AVR and AVL, are obtained in a similar manner (still forgetting the right foot sensor).

To obtain the AVL lead, the left arm electrode sensor is
_____, the other two sensors are negative.   positive

For the AVR lead the _____ arm sensor is positive,   Right
while the remaining sensors are negative.

> NOTE: The right foot sensor is never connected within the
> EKG machine for "Augmented" leads, but it does
> have a sensor wire attached.

> NOTE: AV<u>R</u>—Right arm positive
> AV<u>L</u>—Left arm positive
> AV<u>F</u>—Foot (left foot) positive
> (These augmented limb leads are sometimes called
> the "unipolar" limb leads, stressing the importance
> of the positive electrode.)

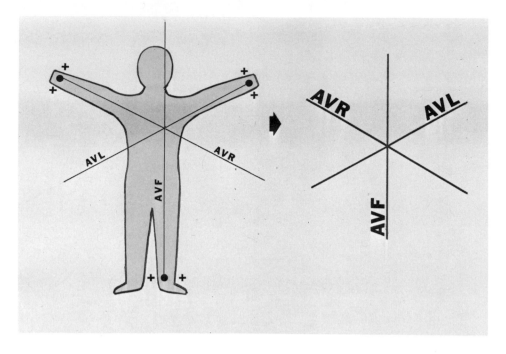

The AVR, AVL, and AVF limb leads intersect at different angles and produce three other intersecting lines of reference.

AVR, AVL, and AVF are also _____ leads.

limb

These leads _____ at 60 degree angles, but the angles differ from those formed by bipolar limb leads I, II, and III.

intersect

Leads AVR, AVL, and AVF intersect at _____ different from leads I, II, and III (and they split the angles formed by I, II, III).

angles

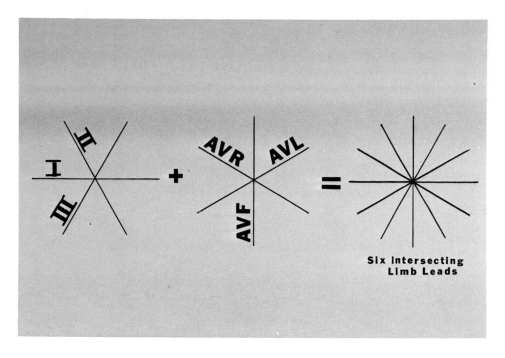

Six Intersecting
Limb Leads

All six limb leads, I, II, III, AVR, AVL, and AVF meet to form six neatly intersecting reference lines which lie in a flat plane on the patient's chest.

The six limb leads are I, II, III, _____, _____, and _____.

AVR, AVL
AVF

If the intersecting leads I, II, and III are superimposed over leads AVR, AVL, and AVF, we have _____ neatly intersecting leads (one every 30 degrees).

six

These limb leads may be visualized as lying in a _____ plane over the patient's chest.

flat

NOTE: The flat plane of the limb leads is known as the *frontal* plane, if anyone asks you.

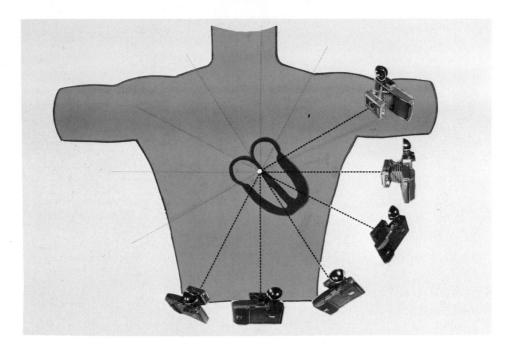

Each limb lead records from a different angle, thus each lead (I, II, III, AVR, AVL, and AVF) is a different view of the same cardiac activity.

The EKG records the same cardiac ———————— in each lead.

activity

The waves look different in the various leads because the electrical activity is monitored from a different ———————— for each lead.

position (or angle)

NOTE: Remember that the electrical activity never changes, but the electrode positions are different for each lead, so the tracing changes slightly in each lead as we change the angle from which we monitor the cardiac activity. Keep in mind the fact that the wave of depolarization is a progressive wave of POSITIVE charges passing down the interior of the myocardial cells. If a depolarization wave moves toward a POSITIVE electrode sensor, this describes a POSITIVE (upward) deflection on the tracing for that particular lead. (A little repetitious, but this point should be stressed.)

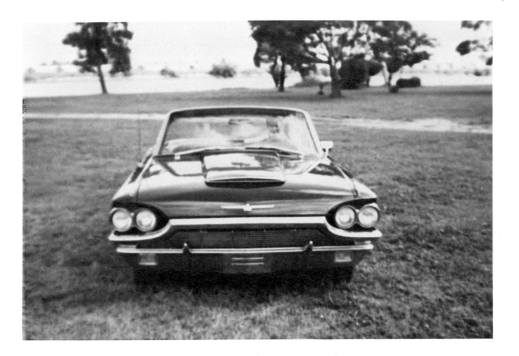

It is important for you to visualize the intersecting limb leads. Why? Can you identify this car?

NOTE: This page sure seems empty doesn't it?

NOTE: Automobile experts are encouraged not to recognize the car for the sake of understanding the analogy.

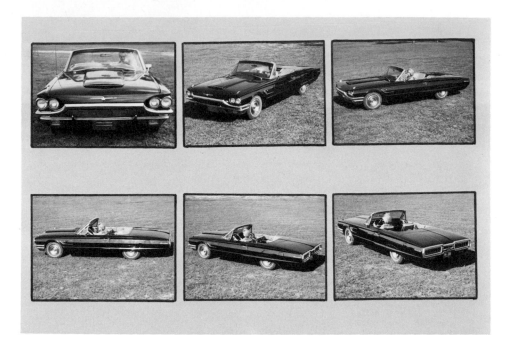

If you observe this same object from six different reference points, you will recognize the car.

NOTE: Observation from six angles is better than one. Thus monitoring cardiac electrical activity from six different angles gives us a much greater perspective. At this point you may take a sip of coffee and relax. Enjoy the automobile display before proceeding. The car, by the way, is a 1965 Thunderbird. The driver is not identified.

NOTE: You can't see the car's back bumper in the picture at top left. But with progressively different views you can tell more about the back bumper (or even the driver if you prefer). Similarly you may not be able to see a certain wave in a given lead, but with six different limb lead positions it should show up better in some leads.

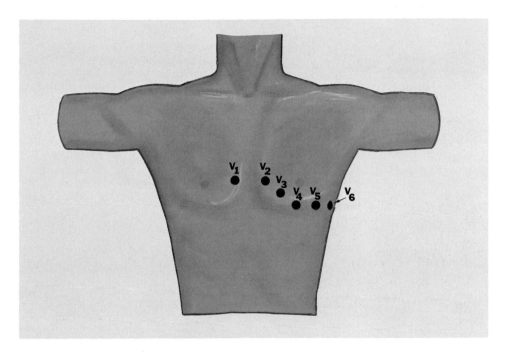

To obtain the six *chest leads*, a positive electrode is placed at six different positions around the chest.

The six chest leads are monitored from six progressively different positions on the _____.

chest

In all of the chest leads, the electrode sensor placed on the chest is considered _____. (This electrode is a suction cup which is moved to a different position on the chest for each different chest lead.)

positive

The chest leads are numbered from V_1 to V_6 and move in successive steps from the patient's _____ to his _____ side. Notice how the chest leads cover the heart in its anatomical position within the chest.

right
left

> NOTE: Because the electrode sensor for the chest leads is always POSITIVE, a depolarization wave moving toward a given chest sensor produces a POSITIVE (upward) deflection in that chest lead on the EKG tracing.

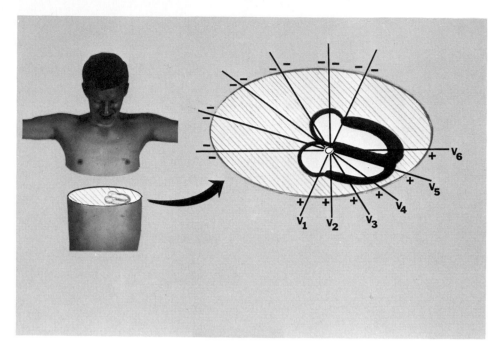

The chest leads* are projected through the AV Node towards the patient's back, which is the negative end of each chest lead.

The skin sensor for each of the chest leads is always considered _____ (positive or negative).

positive

If leads V_1 through V_6 are assumed to be the spokes of a wheel, the center of the wheel is the _____.

AV Node

Lead V_2 describes a straight line from the front to the _____ of the patient. The patient's back is negative in V_2.

back

NOTE: The plane of the chest leads cuts the body into top and bottom halves and is called the *horizontal* plane.

*The chest leads (also called the "precordial" leads) were introduced by Dr. F. N. Wilson.

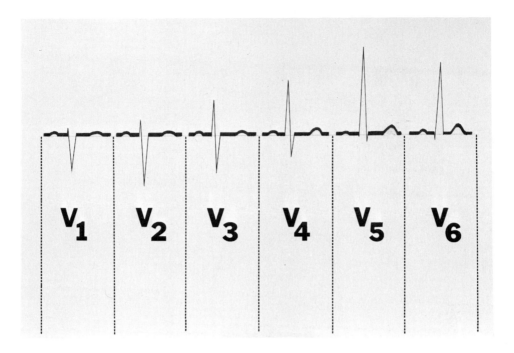

The EKG tracing will thus show progressive changes from V_1 to V_6.

NOTE: When observing the chest leads from V_1 to V_6, one will notice gradual changes in all the waves (as the position of each lead changes).

Considering chest lead V_1, the QRS complex is mainly
_____ (positive or negative) normally (i.e.,   negative
mainly above or below baseline).

In chest lead V_6 the QRS complex is usually
_____ (positive or negative).   positive

This means that the (positive) wave of ventricular
depolarization (represented by the QRS complex) is moving
_____ (toward or away from) the POSITIVE chest   toward
electrode of lead V_6. (Make certain that you understand this
concept. If not, check page 11.)

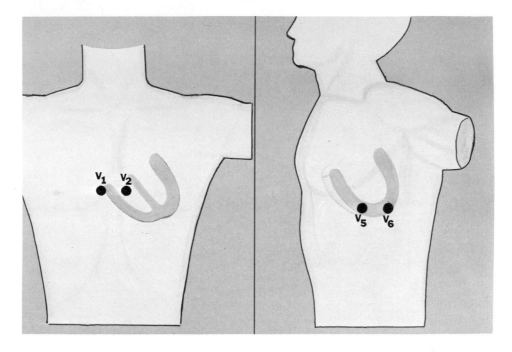

Leads V_1 and V_2 are placed over the right side of the heart, while V_5 and V_6 are over the left side of the heart.

Leads V_1 and V_2 are called the "_____" chest leads.

right

The two leads over the left side of the heart are
_____ and _____ (and are called the "left" chest leads).

V_5 and V_6

A depolarization wave moving toward the (positive) chest electrode in lead V_6 will cause an _____ deflection on the tracing.

upward
(or positive)

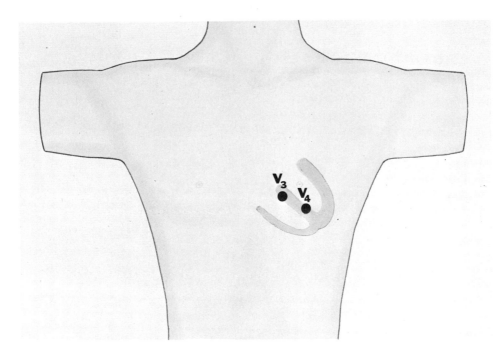

Leads V₃ and V₄ are located over the interventricular septum.

Leads V₃ and V₄ are located generally over the
interventricular _____.   septum

> NOTE: The interventricular septum is a common wall
> shared by the Right and Left Ventricle. In this area the
> His Bundle divides into Right and Left Bundle Branches.

Considering lead V₃, the chest electrode is said to be
_____ (positive or negative).   positive

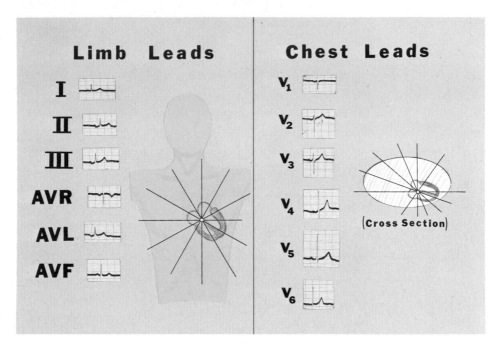

On a standard EKG mounting there are the six chest leads and six limb leads. This is the 12 lead electrocardiogram.

The standard EKG has six chest leads usually mounted in progressive order V_1 to _____.

V_6

The limb leads all lie in a plane which can be _____ over the chest of the patient. (This is the *frontal* plane.)

visualized

The chest leads progressively encircle the heart in the _____ plane.

horizontal

NOTE: The chest leads form the *horizontal* plane which cuts the body into top and bottom halves.

1. Rate

2. Rhythm

3. Axis

4. Hypertrophy

5. Infarction

In the actual reading of an EKG you must check five general areas.

The most valuable areas to be considered in EKG interpretation are *Rate, Rhythm, Axis, Hypertrophy,* and *Infarction.* All of these areas are equally important, so there are no blanks to fill in here.

NOTE: Take a moment and examine page 280. This simple methodology is to become your routine. *Before* you begin each chapter, become familiar with its summary (page 280), so while you assimilate each chapter an "aha!" will light up in your brain as your *understanding* evolves, for this is the foundation of your *knowledge.*

Ready?

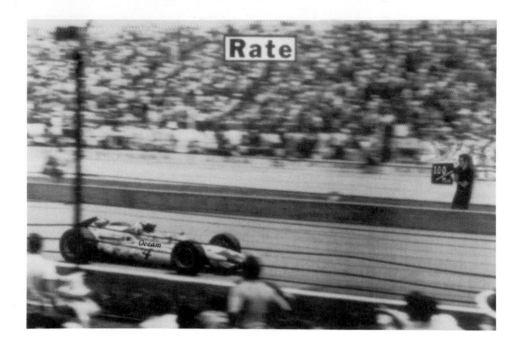

When reading an EKG you should first consider the rate.

NOTE: The sign in this picture is not informing the driver about the rate of his car. The man holding that sign is a physician who has been monitoring the driver's transmitted EKG. The sign is informing the driver about his heart rate (he's a little excited).

When examining an EKG you should first determine the _____.   rate

The rate is read as cycles per _____ .   minute

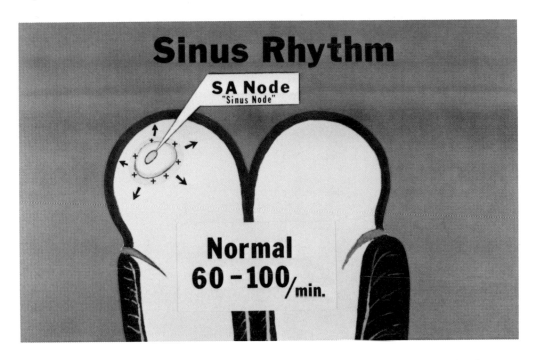

The SA Node (Sinus Node) normally acts as pacemaker and sets the heart rate of 60 to 100 beats per minute.

The normal cardiac rate is set by the _____.   SA Node

The SA Node is located within the upper-posterior wall of
the right _____.   atrium

The SA Node is the normal cardiac pace- _____.   maker

> NOTE: The SA Node (or "Sinus Node") is the heart's
> normal pacemaker, so its normal, regular rhythm is called
> a *Sinus Rhythm.*

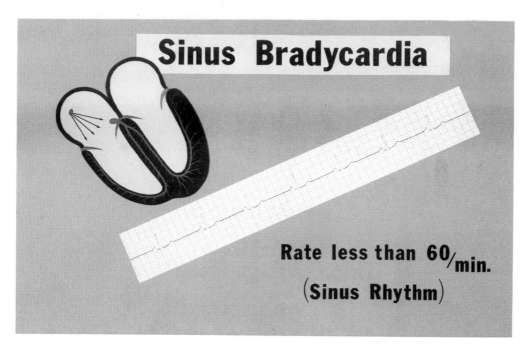

When the SA Node (Sinus Node) paces the heart at a rate slower than 60 per minute, this is called *Sinus Bradycardia*.

A rhythm originating in the heart's normal pacemaker, the SA Node, with a rate less than 60 per minute is called a Sinus _____.

Bradycardia

Sinus Bradycardia is present if a rate of less than one beat per second is produced by the SA _____.

Node

NOTE: Although the cycles are widely separated, the P, QRS, and T waves are still grouped together, but there are longer spans between cycles. Sinus Bradycardia is a slower-than-normal Sinus Rhythm.

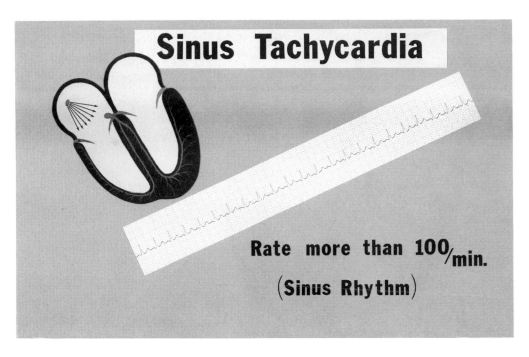

When the SA Node (Sinus Node) paces the heart at a rate greater than 100 per minute, this is called *Sinus Tachycardia.*

NOTE: A faster-than-normal Sinus Rhythm is called Sinus Tachycardia.

A rhythm originating in the SA Node is called Sinus Tachycardia when the rate is greater than _____ per minute.

100

The Sinus Node is another name for the SA Node which is the heart's normal _____.

pacemaker

NOTE: There are other areas (foci) of the heart which have the capability of pacing when needed (see next page).

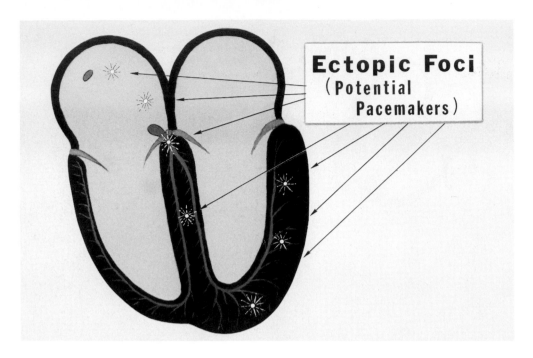

Ectopic Foci
(Potential
Pacemakers)

Other areas of the heart have the ability to pace if the normal (SA Node) pacemaking mechanism fails.

If the SA Node does not function normally, there are foci* of _____ pacemakers available to assume the pace-setting activity.

potential

> NOTE: Because these focal centers of potential pacemaking activity originate in other areas of the heart, they are referred to as "ectopic" foci. An ectopic focus will assume pacing responsibility if it senses a failure of the SA Node to pace.

Ectopic foci of potential pacemakers are in the _____, ventricles, and the AV Junction (the region where the AV Node joins the His Bundle).

atria

Under normal conditions these ectopic foci of potential pacemakers are electrically quiet and do not _____. (That's why we call them "potential" pacemakers.)

function (or operate, etc.)

*Foci is the plural of "focus," so called because each is a focal concentration of cells which can initiate and maintain regular pacemaking stimuli.

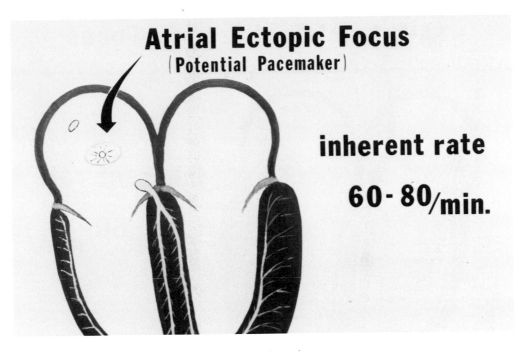

The atria have ectopic foci of potential pacemakers, any one of which may assume pacemaking activity at its "inherent" rate of about 60 to 80/minute if the SA Node fails.

NOTE: Remember *foci* refers to more than one focus.

If the SA Node fails, an atrial ectopic _____ may assume pacing responsibility.

focus (pacemaker)

When an atrial ectopic focus then assumes pacing responsibility, it usually discharges at its "inherent" rate of 60 to _____ /minute, which is very close to the normal rate set by the SA Node.

80

NOTE: You may read or hear the term "focus of automaticity" which implies that foci can automatically emit a series of regular pacing impulses.

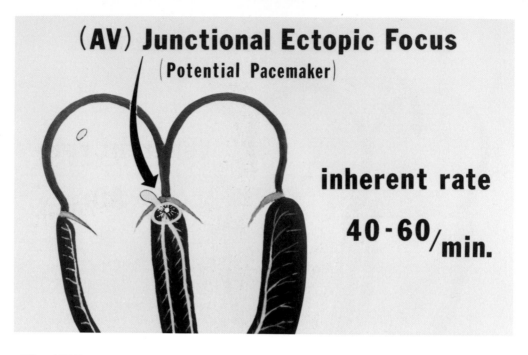

(AV) Junctional Ectopic Focus
(Potential Pacemaker)

inherent rate

40-60/min.

The AV Junction (see NOTE) has ectopic foci of potential pacemakers, any of which will pace at its "inherent" rate of 40 to 60/minute if the usual regular stimulus which normally comes down from the atria is *not* present.

NOTE: The AV Junction is the area where the AV Node meets the His Bundle.

An ectopic _____ in the AV Junction begins to pace only if the normal stimulus from the atria (via the AV Node) is absent.

focus

When a Junctional ectopic focus assumes pacing at its "inherent" rate of 40 to 60 per _____, this is called an *idiojunctional** rhythm.

minute

*The prefix "idio-" is of Greek origin and means "one's own".

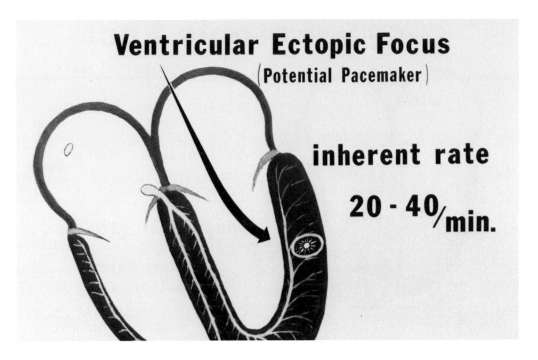

Ventricular Ectopic Focus
(Potential Pacemaker)

inherent rate
20 - 40/min.

The ventricles also have ectopic foci of potential pacemakers, any one of which will assume pacing at its "inherent" rate of 20 to 40/minute if the usual stimuli (which normally come down from above) are absent.

The _____ also have ectopic foci of potential pacemakers.

ventricles

A ventricular pacemaker (focus) assumes a pace of _____ to _____ /minute when the normal stimuli coming from above are absent.

20 40

When a ventricular ectopic focus paces the heart at its _____ rate of 20 to 40 per minute, this is an *idioventricular* rhythm.

inherent

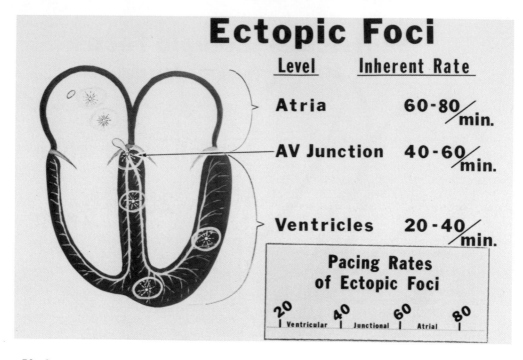

If the normal pacing activity of the SA Node fails, an ectopic focus in the atria, AV Junction, or in the ventricles can assume the pacemaking responsibility at its own inherent rate.

In case of failure of SA Node pacing, an atrial ectopic focus will pace the heart at its inherent rate of _____ to 80 per minute, but a focus in the AV Junction will pace at its slower inherent rate of 40–60/minute.

60

The ventricles can be paced by a ventricular ectopic focus at its inherent rate of _____ to _____ per minute, if no pacemaking activity from above can be detected.

20 40

NOTE: In emergency or certain pathological conditions the ectopic foci in any of these three areas may suddenly discharge at a rapid rate. The rapid rate (150 to 250/min.) is the same for foci in the atria, AV Junction, and ventricles.

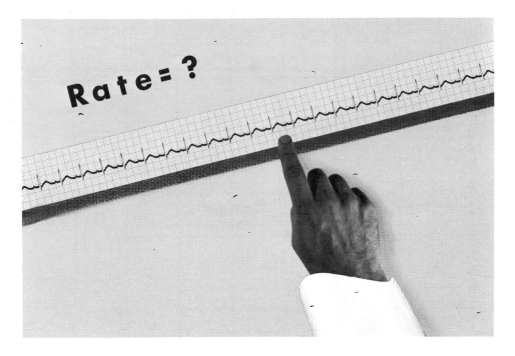

Our main objective is to rapidly determine the rate.

After finishing this chapter you will be able to determine
the _____ rapidly.   rate

No special devices, calculators, rulers or awkward
mathematical computations are needed in order to
_____ the rate.   determine

> NOTE: In emergency situations you will probably not be
> able to find your calculator. THROW IT AWAY!

Observation alone can tell us the _____.   rate

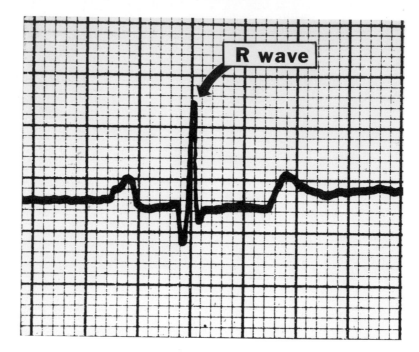

First: find a specific R wave that falls on a heavy black line.

To calculate *rate* you should first look at the _____ waves.   R

Now find one which peaks on a heavy black _____.   line

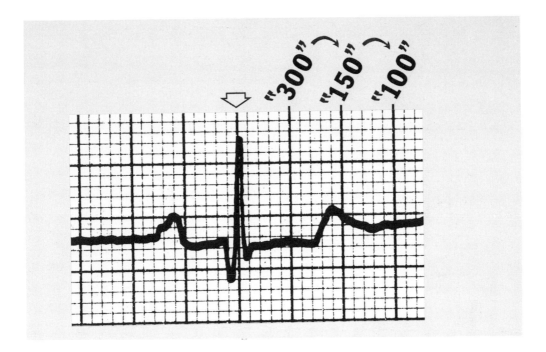

Next: Count off "300, 150, 100" for each heavy black line that follows, naming each one as shown. Memorize these numbers.

An R wave falls on a heavy black line . . . the next heavy
black line is called " _____ ". . . followed by   300
" _____, _____ " for the next two heavy lines.   150, 100

NOTE: The line which the R wave peaks upon has no
name. We only name the lines that follow.

The three lines following the line where the R wave falls
are named " _____, _____, _____ " in   300, 150, 100
succession.

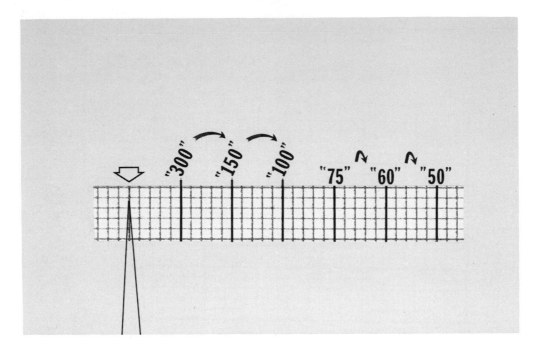

Then: Count off the next three lines after "300, 150, 100" as "75, 60, 50."

The next three lines after "300, 150, 100" are called " _____,   75
60, and 50."

Remember the next three lines together as " _____,   75
_____, _____." Name them as you go.   60, 50

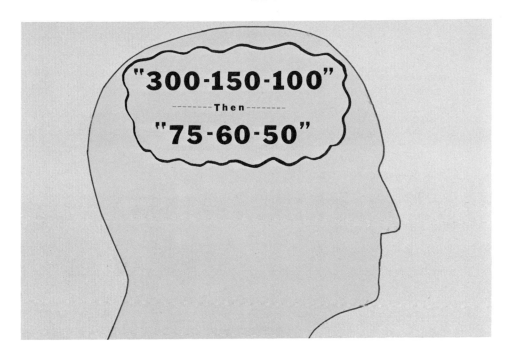

Now: Memorize these triplicates until they are second nature. Make certain you can *say* the triplicates without using the picture.

These triplicates, "300, 150, 100" and "75, 60, 50" must be
_____.   memorized

Be able to name the lines following that one on which an R wave _____; it is easy to remember them as   peaks triplicates.

Do not count those lines which follow—name them with the
_____ as you go.   triplicates

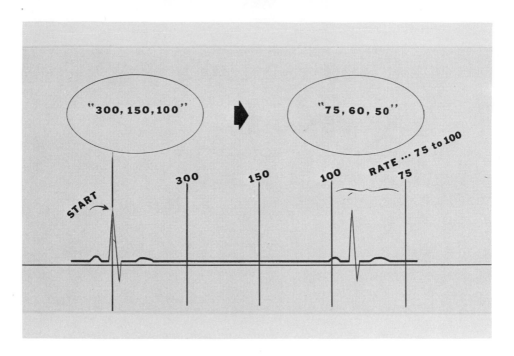

Where the next R wave falls determines the rate. It is that simple.

Find an R wave peaked upon a heavy line, then look for the next ___ _____.

R   wave

Where the next R wave falls gives the _____. There is no mathematical computation necessary.

rate

If the R wave falls on "75" the rate is 75 per _____.

minute

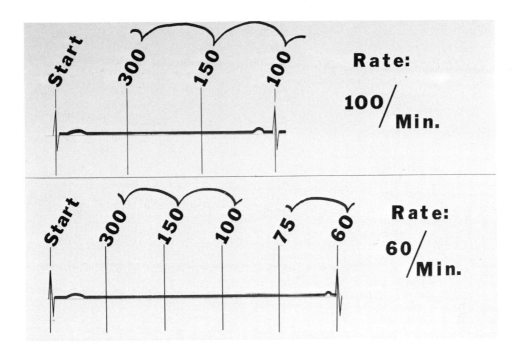

Knowing the triplicates "300, 150, 100" and "75, 60, 50," you can merely look at an EKG and tell the approximate rate.

The triplicates are: first " _____, _____, _____."
                      then " _____, _____, _____."

                                                    300, 150, 100
                                                    75, 60, 50

By merely naming the lines using
_____, you can immediately identify   triplicates
the rate.

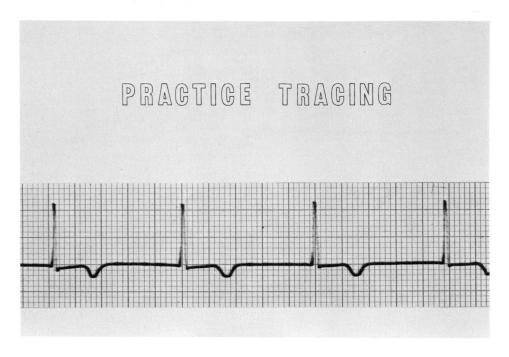

This is the EKG tracing from a patient with a heart rate slower than his usual rate. Determine the rate.

The rate in the above tracing is about _____ cycles per minute.

60

If you were told that this rate originated in an ectopic focus (pacemaker), you would probably suspect the _____ (by the rate alone).

AV Junction

NOTE: This is indeed a rhythm originating in the AV Junction, and that is why you can't see any P waves.

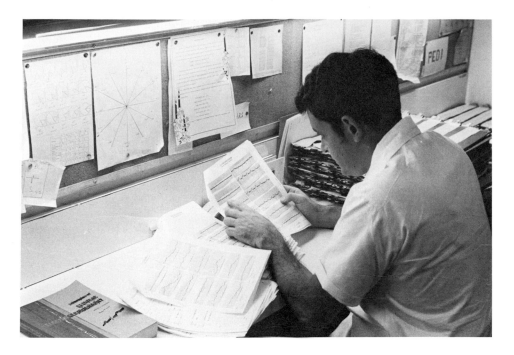

You do not need to depend on mathematical calculations, because the rate can be determined very easily by simple observation.

You can rapidly determine the rate on an EKG tracing by
_____ alone.   observation

There is no need to depend on annoying math or calculators
to determine the _____.   rate

> NOTE: You will always have your brain with you (until
> that time when brain transplants are done and you may
> have someone else's brain). Just remember to name the
> lines that follow the "R wave line" using the triplicates,
> and say "300, 150, 100" then "75, 60, 50."

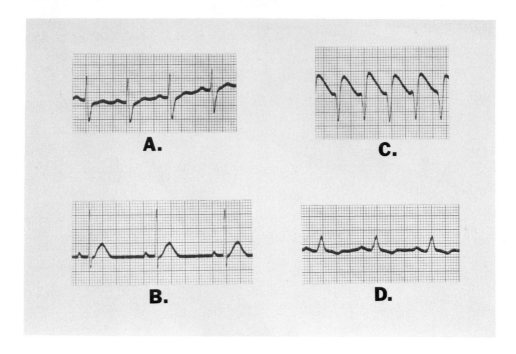

Give the approximate rates of the above EKG tracings.

A. _____   100

B. _____   60

C. _____   150 or so

D. _____   75

NOTE: As you have no doubt discovered for yourself, any prominent wave (like the S wave in example C.) can be used to determine the rate.

The distance between the heavy black lines represents 1/300 min.

So two 1/300 min. units = 2/300 min. = 1/150 min.(or 150/min. rate)

and three 1/300 units = 3/300 = 1/100 min.(or 100/min. rate)

There is a logical explanation for the seemingly unusual rate denominations for the heavy black lines.

NOTE: The unit (duration) of time between two heavy black lines is 1/300th minute.

The number of time units between five consecutive heavy black lines is _____.

4

So this represents 4/300 minute or a rate of _____ per minute.

75

Therefore if a heart contracts 75 times/minute, there will be a span equivalent to the distance between five heavy black lines between _____ complexes.

QRS

NOTE: Reasonable instructors should not require students to master this page. As author, I have not personally memorized the material on this page. Let's keep it simple.

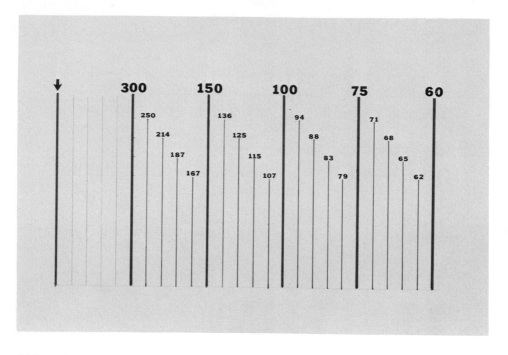

Although memorization of the fine divisions is a tremendous undertaking, more exact determination of rates is possible.

NOTE: It is admittedly a great task to memorize the fine subdivisions, but it is convenient to have this information (see page 281) for your reference should you need it.

NOTE: For rates less than sixty see the next few pages for a very simple method of rate determination.

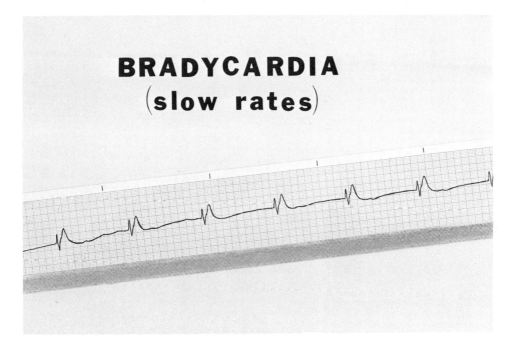

BRADYCARDIA
(slow rates)

For very slow rhythms we offer an easy method to determine the rate rapidly.

Slow rates are called _____.   Bradycardia

For very _____ rhythms you can use another method to   slow
determine the rate.

> NOTE: The triplicates give us a very large range of rates.
> "300, 150, 100" and "75, 60, 50" means that you can
> determine rates ranging from 300 to 50. Bradycardia
> means a rate less than 60 per minute.

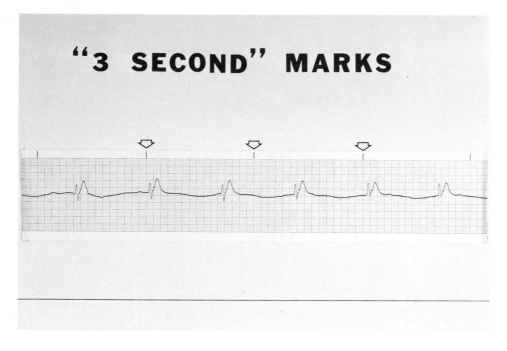

"3 SECOND" MARKS

At the top of the EKG tracing there are small marks which signify "three second" intervals.

There are small marks above the _____ portion of the EKG tracing. Find a strip of EKG tracing and examine it.

graph

These marks are called "three second" _____ marks.

interval

NOTE: Some EKG paper has 3 second intervals marked with a black dot, circle, arrow, vertical line, etc.

When the EKG machine is running, the span of paper between two of these (3 second interval) marks passes under the stylus needle in _____ _____.

three seconds

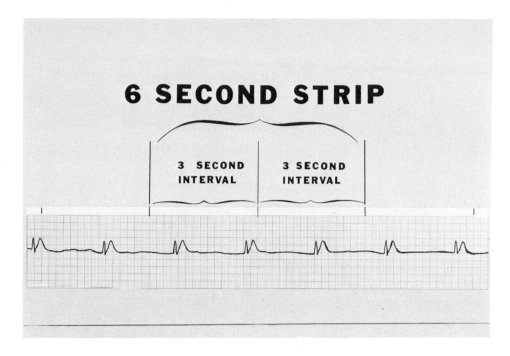

Taking two of the three second intervals, we have a 6 second strip.

NOTE: A three second interval is obviously the distance between two consecutive three second interval marks.

Taking two of the three second intervals gives us a
_____ second strip.   six

This six second strip represents the amount of _____   paper
used by the machine in six seconds (one tenth of a minute).

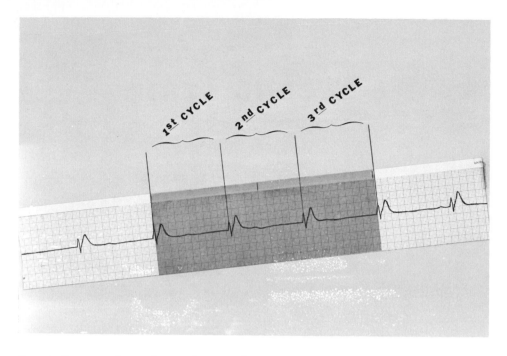

Count the number of complete cycles (R wave-to-R wave may be used to represent the length of one cycle) in this strip. With very slow rates there will be few cycles.

The length of a cardiac _____ can be measured from a specific wave until the wave is repeated again.

cycle

So, R wave to _____ wave gives one cycle (in length).

R

Count the number of cycles in the six second _____.

strip

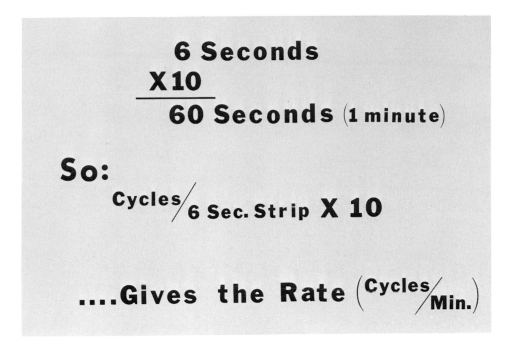

6 Seconds
X 10
_____
60 Seconds (1 minute)

So:

Cycles⁄6 Sec. Strip **X 10**

....Gives the Rate (Cycles⁄Min.)

The rate is obtained by multiplying the number of cycles in the six second strip by 10.

Ten of the 6 second strips equals one _____ (time) recorded on EKG.

minute

The number of cycles per minute is the _____.

rate

So cycles per six second strip multiplied by _____ equals the rate.

ten

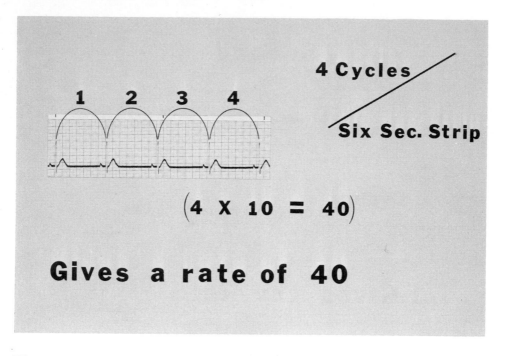

Gives a rate of 40

Place a zero on the right of the number of cycles/six second strip and you have the rate.

For very slow rates or _____ first find   bradycardia
a six second strip.

. . . count the number of _____ in this strip.   cycles

. . . and multiply by _____ to get the rate.   ten

NOTE: Multiplying by ten may be done by placing a zero on the right side of the number of cycles per six second strip. For instance, 5 cycles (per six second strip) gives a rate of 50.

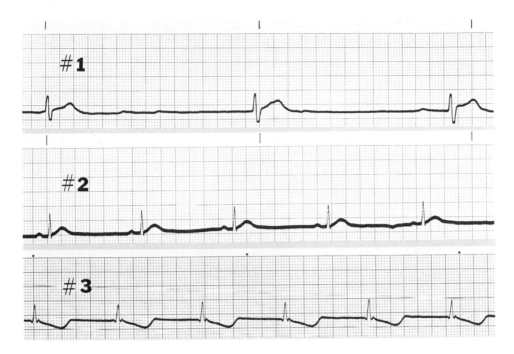

Give the approximate rates of these EKG's.

Rates: No. 1 ＿＿ per minute   20
        No. 2 ＿＿ per minute   45
        No. 3 ＿＿ per minute   50

NOTE: The general, average rates of irregular rhythms also may be determined using this method. Obtain some EKG tracings and amaze yourself at how easily you can now determine the rate.

NOTE: Review *Rate* by turning to the **P**ersonal **Q**uick **R**eference **S**heets at the end of this book (pages 280 and 281).

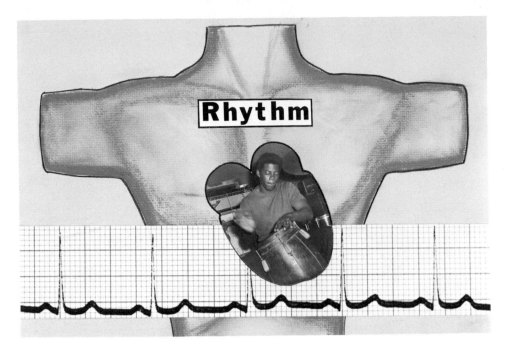

The EKG provides the most accurate means for identifying cardiac arrhythmias (abnormal rhythms) which can be easily diagnosed by understanding the electro-physiology of the heart.

_____ literally means without rhythm; however, we use it to denote abnormal rhythm, or breaks in the regularity of a normal rhythm.

Arrhythmia

The _____ records the electrical phenomena of the heart which may not be seen, felt, or heard on physical examination, and therefore provides a very accurate means for determining rhythm changes.

EKG

NOTE: To understand the arrhythmias you must first be familiar with the normal electrophysiology of the heart (i.e., the normal pathway of electrical conduction).

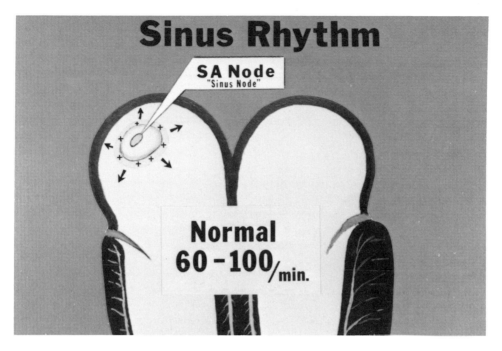

The pacemaker impulse from the SA Node (Sinus Node) spreads through both atria as a wave of depolarization.

It is the _____ which initiates the stimulus for pacemaking activity.

SA Node
(Sinus Node)

The SA Node sends out regular impulses (60 to 100/minute) which cause the atria to _____.

contract

The wave of stimulation called
_____ spreads out from the SA Node in wave fashion and describes a P wave on the EKG.

depolarization

NOTE: The SA Node is the "Sino-Atrial" Node, so impulses originating from this node are often identified by the stem "Sinus" or "Sino" as in regular Sinus Rhythm. It is also called the Sinus Node.

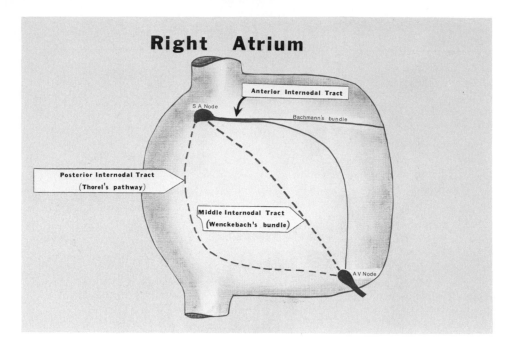

The atrial conduction system consists of three specialized conduction pathways

Three general atrial conduction pathways are known today; the anterior, middle, and _____ internodal tracts.

posterior

The posterior internodal tract is known as _____ pathway.

Thorel's

This page serves as a reference, for specific pathological conditions involving these preferential conduction pathways have not as yet been described, but certainly will in the future. For now, it suffices to recognize their existence.

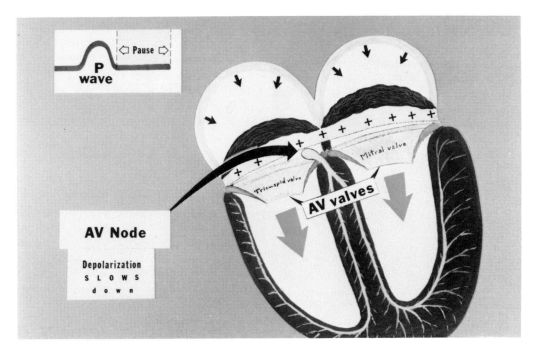

The electrical stimulus (from the atria) reaches the AV Node, and then there is a brief pause while the stimulus slowly penetrates through the AV Node.

As the impulse from atrial depolarization slowly makes its way through the AV Node, there is a _____.   pause

> NOTE: The AV Node is named for its position between the
> Atria and the Ventricles (thus "AV").
> The **AV Node has no foci** of potential pacemakers.

This pause during which there is no cardiac electrical activity is represented by the flat piece of baseline between the _____ wave and the QRS complex.   P

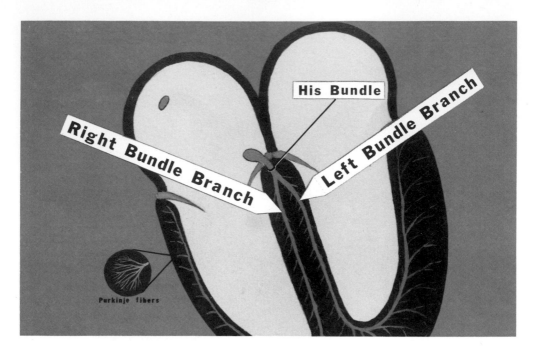

Once depolarization has penetrated through the AV Node completely, this electrical stimulus proceeds rapidly through the His Bundle, the Bundle Branches, and the terminal Purkinje fibers to depolarize the ventricular myocardium.

Once the stimulus has penetrated through the AV Node, it continues rapidly through the His ⎯⎯⎯⎯⎯.   Bundle

From the His Bundle the impulse is rapidly conducted down the Left and Right Bundle ⎯⎯⎯⎯⎯⎯⎯, through the   Branches
terminal Purkinje fibers and into the myocardial cells.

NOTE: The impulse of depolarization passes slowly through the AV Node, but it proceeds very rapidly within the His Bundle, Bundle Branches, and Purkinje fibers to the myocardial cells which depolarize and produce a QRS complex on the EKG.

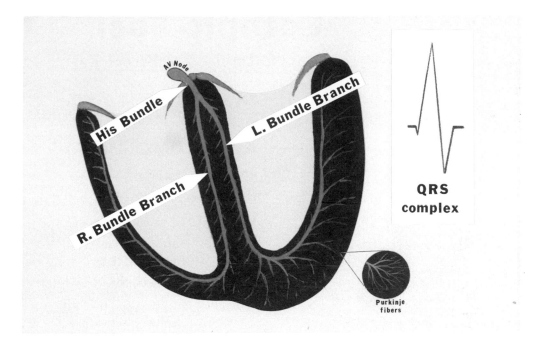

This ventricular conduction system below the AV Node is made of specialized nervous tissue which carries the electrical stimulus (depolarization) rapidly.

The ventricular conduction system
(His Bundle—Bundle Branches—Purkinje fibers) is made of
specialized _____ tissue.   nervous

This nervous tissue conducts electrical _____   impulses
rapidly.

NOTE: I would like to stress the fact that this specialized
nervous tissue carries electrical impulses to the ventricles
quite rapidly. Cardiac muscle itself conducts bio-electrical
charges more slowly, therefore it is easy to recognize
pathological impulses that originate outside the ventricular
conduction system (they are slower on EKG).

NOTE: It is only the depolarization of the ventricular
myocardial cells which produces the QRS. The passage of
depolarization through the AV Node and the ventricular
conduction system below is NOT recorded on EKG.

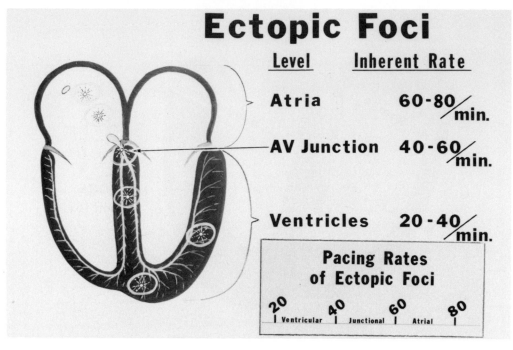

Ectopic Foci

Level	Inherent Rate
Atria	60-80/min.
AV Junction	40-60/min.
Ventricles	20-40/min.

Pacing Rates of Ectopic Foci

20   40   60   80

| Ventricular | Junctional | Atrial |

There are ectopic foci of potential pacemakers (in both atria, in the AV Junction, and in both ventricles) which can assume pacing responsibility if normal pacing fails.

NOTE: The AV Junction is located at the junction of the AV Node and the His Bundle.

Ectopic foci of potential pacemakers exist in the atria, ventricles, and the AV _____.

Junction

There are ectopic foci of potential pacemakers which can assume _____ responsibility if normal pacing activity fails.

pacing

Because these potential pacemakers are not part of the SA Node, and they are found in other regions of the heart, they are called _____ (abnormal location) foci.

ectopic

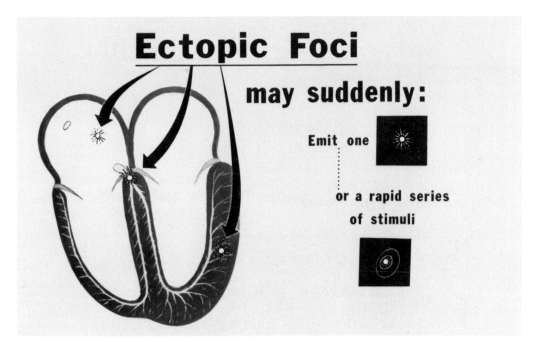

Ectopic Foci

may suddenly:

Emit one

or a rapid series
of stimuli

These ectopic foci occasionally emit an electrical impulse spontaneously, or a series of rapid impulses may suddenly erupt.

The ectopic focus is an area in the atria, AV Junction, or ventricles which can emit electrical

_____.

stimuli
(or impulses)

An ectopic focus may suddenly discharge one or a _____ of rapid impulses in a pathological or emergency situation.

series

NOTE: All the arrhythmias may be easily mastered simply by understanding the normal electro-physiology (conduction) of the heart and realizing the existence of ectopic foci. As each of the arrhythmias is presented, visualize what is taking place in the heart (electrically), and interpretation of the tracing becomes an easy matter. Do not memorize patterns. _Lasting knowledge results from understanding._

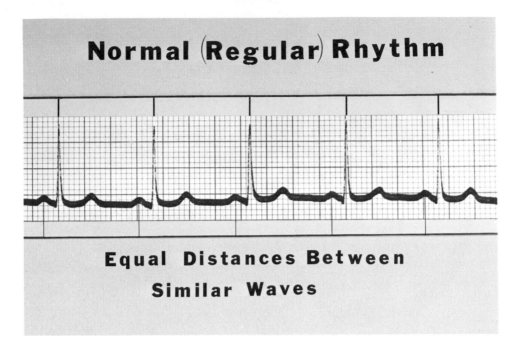

There is a consistent distance between similar waves with a normal ("regular") cardiac rhythm.

The normal rhythm of the heart is said to be
_____.   regular

The distance between similar _____ is always the   waves
same in a classical regular rhythm.

> NOTE: The normal rhythm is often referred to as a
> "Regular" Sinus Rhythm or "Normal" Sinus Rhythm since
> it originates in the SA Node (Sinus Node).

> NOTE: Like the SA Node, when an ectopic focus is pacing
> (either at a slow or rapid rate), the rhythm is generally
> regular. All healthy pacemakers are characteristically
> regular.

Arrhythmias

Irregular Rhythms

"Escape" and Premature Beats

Rapid Ectopic Rhythms

Heart Blocks

The arrhythmias* may be divided into a few general categories.

NOTE: Although *arrhythmia* means literally "without rhythm," it is used generally to denote any variance from a normal Sinus Rhythm.

NOTE: It is not necessary to memorize our general classification of the arrhythmias. The classification of these four general varieties is intended to help you [Rapidly] recognize the type of pathology by appearance. The underlying mechanisms are basic to the heart's function and quite easy to understand. Lasting knowledge results from understanding.

*Another term: *Dysrhythmia* ("abnormal rhythm") is commonly used in medical literature.

Irregular Rhythms

Sinus Arrhythmia

Wandering Pacemaker

Atrial Fibrillation

Irregular rhythms are usually caused by irregularity of pacing or multiple sources of pacing.

The _____ rhythms are those rhythms with generally inconsistent irregularity.

irregular

> NOTE: Some of these arrhythmias are referred to as "irregularly irregular" since no precise recurring pattern of irregularity can be found.

Sometimes pacemaker foci of different areas of the same chamber(s) are operating at once, producing a very _____ rhythm.

irregular

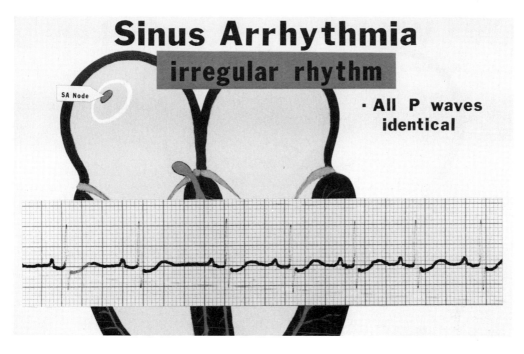

Sinus Arrhythmia
irregular rhythm

SA Node

· All P waves identical

Sinus Arrhythmia is an irregular rhythm related to the phases of respiration (increasing rate with inspiration, decreasing rate with expiration).

In Sinus Arrhythmia the pacemaking impulses originate in the SA Node (thus the prefix "Sinus"). Because all impulses originate in the SA Node, all _____ waves are identical.

P

The pacemaking activity is irregular and is usually linked to inspiration and _____.

expiration

The P-QRS-T waves of each cycle are usually _____ and similar in size and shape, but there is a continuous, gradual rate change: increasing with inspiration and decreasing with expiration.

normal

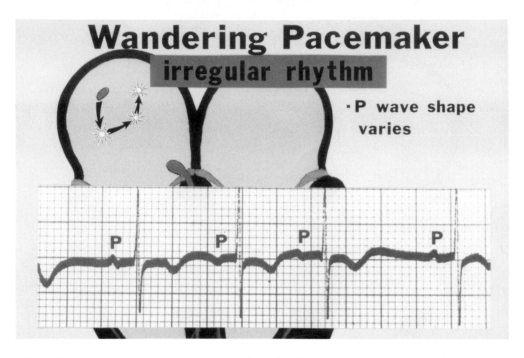

Wandering Pacemaker
irregular rhythm
·P wave shape varies

Wandering Pacemaker is an irregular rhythm caused by pacing discharges from a variety of different atrial foci. It is characterized by P waves of varying shape.

In Wandering Pacemaker the pacemaking _____ wanders from focus to focus.

activity

The resulting rhythm is very _____, and there is no consistent pattern to the rhythm.

irregular

The ____ waves of Wandering Pacemaker are of various shapes, since the pacemaking origin continuously changes location within the atria.

P

NOTE: Should this rhythm exceed a rate of 100 per minute, it is then called *Multifocal Atrial Tachycardia*.

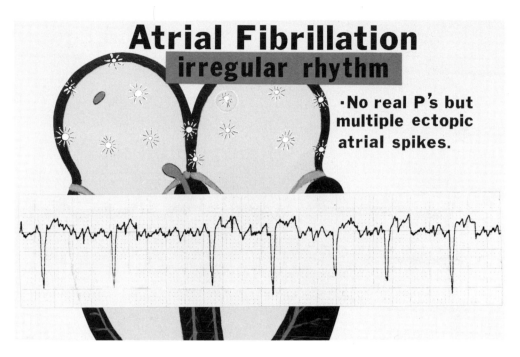

Atrial Fibrillation
irregular rhythm

·No real P's but multiple ectopic atrial spikes.

Atrial Fibrillation is caused by the continuous, rapid-firing of multiple foci in the atria. No single impulse depolarizes the atria completely, and only an occasional impulse gets through the AV Node to stimulate the ventricles, producing an *irregular ventricular* (QRS) *rhythm.*

Atrial Fibrillation is caused by multiple ectopic _____ in the atria which emit electrical impulses.

foci

Since no single impulse depolarizes both atria, we cannot find any real ____ waves, only a rapid series of tiny, erratic spikes on EKG.

P

This is always a totally erratic atrial rhythm, and only random impulses get through the AV Node to initiate a _____ complex. The *irregular ventricular responses* may produce a rapid or slow ventricular rate, but it is always irregular.

QRS

NOTE: It is a good practice to ALWAYS determine and document the general (average) ventricular rate in Atrial Fibrillation (QRS's per 6-second strip times 10).

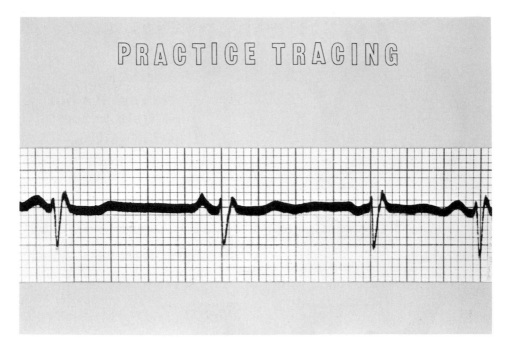

This tracing was monitored from a patent with a very irregular pulse.

In this practice tracing we notice an irregular rhythm in which we can see discernible _____ waves, so we can rule out Atrial Fibrillation.

P

The P waves are not identical, so we can say that this tracing is probably not _____ Arrhythmia.

Sinus

It is most likely a tracing of _____ _____, particularly with P waves of differing shapes.

Wandering Pacemaker

Easy, isn't it?

NOTE: A quick review of the illustrations on pages 87, 88, 89, and 90 will help you grasp and differentiate the irregular rhythms.

"Escape"

and

Premature Beats

"Escape" describes the response (of a focus) to a pause in pacemaking activity. But *Premature Beats* are produced by an ectopic focus discharging spontaneously, causing a beat which appears earlier than expected.

NOTE: By scanning a tracing one can easily notice the obvious breaks in the continuity of the rhythm. Recognizable pauses in the SA Node's pacemaking activity may elicit an "escape" response (discharge) from an ectopic focus. However, "premature" beats are due to the spontaneous discharge of an ectopic focus.

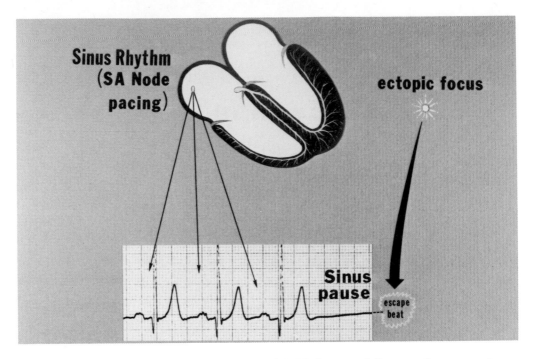

During a Sinus Rhythm, an unhealthy SA Node may fail to produce a pacing stimulus (Sinus Block), so this "pause" elicits a response from an impatient focus producing an *Escape Beat*.

When an unhealthy _____ fails to emit a normal, regular stimulus (Sinus Block), the heart remains temporarily silent.

SA Node

On the EKG a failure of an unhealthy SA Node to pace is seen as a "pause" (flat area of baseline) which is free of _____.

waves

> NOTE: Sinus Block causes "Sinus Pause" during a Sinus Rhythm. On EKG a Sinus Pause is very obvious since it breaks the continuity of a regular rhythm on the tracing.

> NOTE: After such a pause of cardiac non-activity, an ectopic focus may "escape" (respond) by discharging an Escape Beat*. The temporarily blocked SA Node eventually resumes pacing, but if SA Node pacing is "arrested", then an ectopic focus will have to assume pacing responsibility.

*Under certain conditions a marked, abrupt slowing of the Sinus Rhythm can elicit an Escape Beat.

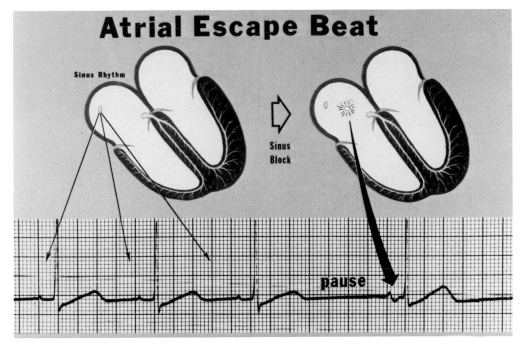

Atrial Escape Beat

A pause in the SA Node pacing may induce an atrial ectopic focus to "escape" to fire an *Atrial Escape Beat*; after depolarizing the atria, the stimulus is then conducted through the AV Node to the ventricles.

Because foci in all areas know that they must be
_____ regularly, they grow impatient when   stimulated
a pause in pacing appears.

An atrial ectopic _____ then "escapes" to emit an   focus
electrical impulse of its own to stimulate the electrically
quiet heart.

When an *atrial* ectopic focus discharges after a silent pause
(from Sinus Block) of one unpaced cycle, the response is
called an Atrial _____ Beat, and because this P wave   Escape
originates ectopically, it usually does not look like the other
P waves (but a normal QRS response follows).

NOTE: If the atrial ectopic focus attains pacemaking
status, this becomes an Atrial Escape *Rhythm*
(rate: 60–80/min.).

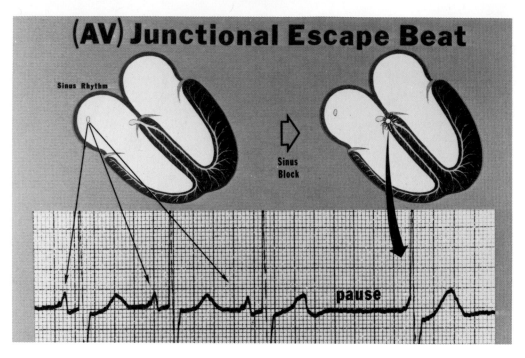

(AV) Junctional Escape Beat

After a pause in SA Node pacing, an *(AV) Junctional Escape Beat* may originate in a focus within the AV Junction and stimulate the ventricles via the ventricular conduction system yielding a normal QRS.

If the SA Node is temporarily blocked, it fails to deliver a
_____ stimulus, so a Sinus Pause is produced on   pacing
EKG. This pause may elicit a Junctional Escape Beat from
a Junctional focus.

The Junctional Escape Beat originates in a focus within the
AV Junction, and the impulse follows* the ventricular
conduction system to both _____.   ventricles

This produces a normal appearing QRS _____   complex
because the ventricles are depolarized just as though the
impulse had originated from above.

> NOTE: If the ectopic Junctional focus attains pacemaking
> status, this becomes a Junctional Escape *Rhythm* (also
> called "idiojunctional rhythm") at its inherent rate of 40 to
> 60/minute.

*Occasionally the Junctional focus may produce an *inverted* P wave (by retrograde atrial stimulation
from below) which occurs just before or just after a QRS of ectopic Junctional origin.

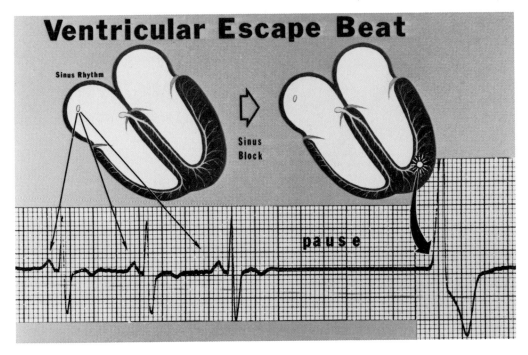

Ventricular Escape Beat

A *Ventricular Escape Beat* originates in a ventricular ectopic focus, producing an enormous ventricular complex after a slightly longer pause in pacing activity.

The Ventricular Escape Beat originates in a ventricular _____ focus which fires an impulse because of an absence of cardiac activity from above.

ectopic

This ventricular ectopic response, because it originates in a ventricular ectopic focus, yields a typical giant ventricular complex after the _____.

pause

NOTE: Any time a ventricular ectopic focus discharges, a giant ventricular complex records on EKG as the ventricles slowly depolarize. The reason for this enormous ventricular complex will be explained soon.

NOTE: If the ectopic ventricular focus attains pacemaking status, this becomes a Ventricular Escape *Rhythm* (or "idioventricular rhythm") at the rate of 20 to 40/minute.

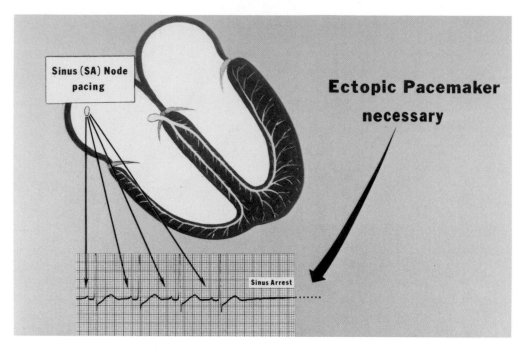

Sinus Arrest occurs when a sick SA Node's pacemaking activity suddenly is "arrested" and does not send out pacemaking stimuli. After the pause of Sinus Arrest, a new pacemaking area (focus) assumes the pacing responsibility.

NOTE: The temporary "pause" of Sinus Block is self descriptive because the SA Node resumes pacing, but with *Sinus Arrest* the SA Node *ceases* pacing.

Sinus Arrest refers to a complete arrest of the pacemaking activity of a sick Sinus _____, producing electrical silence.   Node

Another pacemaker *must* assume pacing acitivity, so an ectopic focus in the atria, AV Junction, or in the ventricles will assume _____ responsibility.   pacemaking

NOTE: Because a new (ectopic) pacemaker assumes the responsibility of pacing, the new pacemaker (ectopic focus) operates at its inherent rate, which is usually slower than the rate of the arrested SA Node.

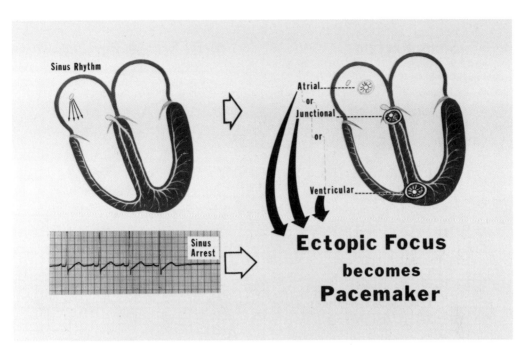

In Sinus Arrest an ectopic focus in the atria, AV Junction, or ventricles "escapes" to assume the pacing responsibility (at its inherent rate).

NOTE: Remember: "escape" is the response of an ectopic focus to a pause of cardiac non-activity. The Escape Rhythms are the heart's backup mechanism in case of Sinus Arrest. So wonderfully designed is the heart!

With Sinus Arrest an atrial ectopic _____ is most likely to "escape" (respond) by initiating an *Atrial Escape Rhythm* at 60 to 80 beats per minute (its inherent rate).

focus

Or a focus in the AV Junction may "escape" to assume pacing responsibility, producing a *Junctional Escape Rhythm* ("idiojunctional rhythm") at 40 to 60 per _____ (its inherent rate).

minute

Or after a long pause, a ventricular ectopic focus may escape (if the foci above don't respond), producing a _____ *Escape Rhythm* ("idioventricular rhythm") at 20 to 40 per minute (its inherent rate).

Ventricular

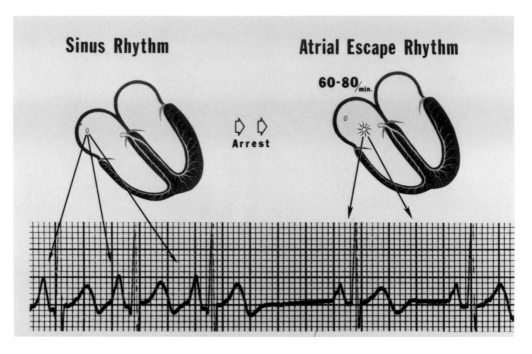

After a Sinus Arrest, an atrial ectopic focus is most likely to "escape" (respond to the absense of pacing), thus initiating an *Atrial Escape Rhythm* at its inherent rate of 60 to 80/minute.

After Sinus Arrest an atrial ectopic _____ is most likely to respond.   focus

So the resulting Atrial Escape Rhythm usually has P waves of slightly different appearance at the (inherent) rate of 60 to 80 per _____.   minute

      NOTE: Also, an atrial ectopic focus will usually have an [inherent] rate that differs from the previous (Sinus) rate (see illustration).

Atrial Escape Rhythm describes the mechanism which initiates the rhythm, and we understand that it is due to an atrial ectopic focus which escapes to assume _____ responsibility.   pacemaking

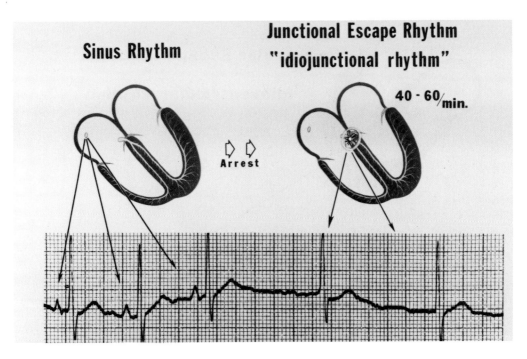

Sometimes an ectopic focus in the AV Junction may "escape" to assume pacing responsibility, producing a *Junctional Escape Rhythm* at its inherent rate of 40 to 60 per minute in the presence of Sinus Arrest.

Sometimes with Sinus Arrest a Junctional
_____ focus will "escape" to assume pacemaking   ectopic
responsibility.

This focus initiates a Junctional Escape Rhythm which
produces normal appearing QRS's without _____ waves* at   P
its inherent rate of 40 to 60 per minute.

This is also called an "idiojunctional rhythm" which
describes a Junctional ectopic focus pacing at its inherent
_____, but should it "accelerate" above the inherent   rate
rate, this becomes an *Accelerated Idiojunctional Rhythm.*

*Occasionally *inverted* (retrograde) P's may occur just before or after a QRS of Junctional origin.

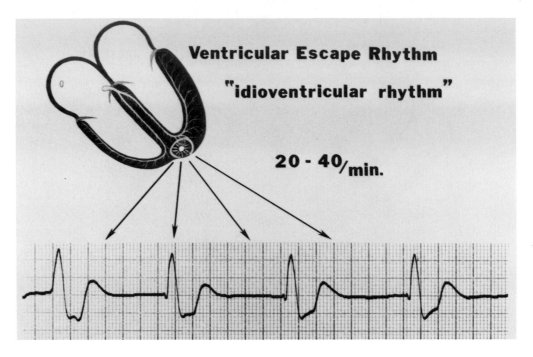

After a Sinus Arrest if higher level foci don't respond, a ventricular ectopic focus may escape to initiate a *Ventricular Escape Rhythm* pacing the heart at its inherent rate of 20 to 40 per minute.

With Sinus Arrest, the atrial and Junctional foci may be faulty, so a _____ ectopic focus escapes   ventricular
to assume pacing responsibility.

The resulting Ventricular Escape Rhythm originates in a ventricular ectopic focus, so it produces enormous ventricular complexes at the rate of 20 to 40 per
_____.   minute

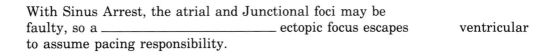

NOTE: This so-called "idioventricular rhythm" is due to a ventricular ectopic focus pacing the heart at its inherent rate.* This rate may be so slow that unconsciousness results (Stokes-Adams Syndrome), making it imperative that the patient be attended to maintain an open airway.

NOTE: You should quickly review the illustrations on pages 91 to 100 to etch this understanding in your permanent memory.

*Should this "accelerate" above the inherent rate, it becomes an *Accelerated Idioventricular Rhythm*.

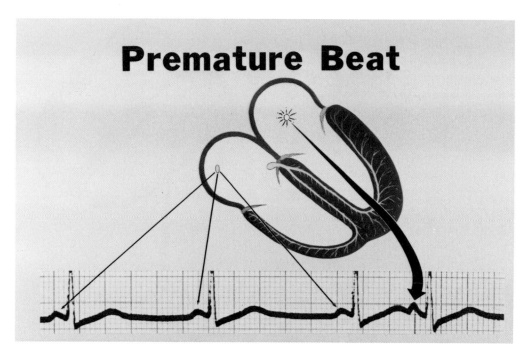

Premature Beat

A *Premature Beat* originates in an ectopic focus which suddenly discharges, producing a beat which appears earlier than expected in the rhythm (the first three cycles in the illustration demonstrate a normal Sinus Rhythm).

Premature beats, like premature babies, occur _____ than expected in a rhythm.

earlier

A premature beat originates in an ectopic _____ (in the atria, AV Junction, or ventricles) which suddenly discharges.

focus

NOTE: A premature beat may be normal in appearance, or it may be an unusual form, but it always appears suddenly, very early in the cycle.

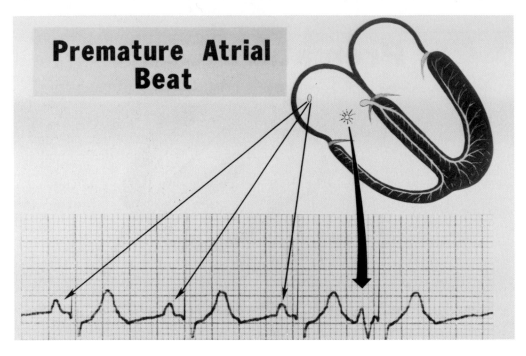

A *Premature Atrial Beat* originates suddenly in an atrial ectopic focus and produces an abnormal P wave earlier than expected.

A Premature Atrial Beat originates in an ectopic focus in
an atrium and appears much earlier than the normal
_____ wave on EKG.

P

A Premature Atrial Beat will not appear like the other P
waves in the same lead because this impulse does not
originate in the _____.

SA Node

This ectopic impulse depolarizes the atria in a manner
similar to the normal impulse, so the AV Node picks up and
transmits the impulse just as if it were a normal _____
wave.

P

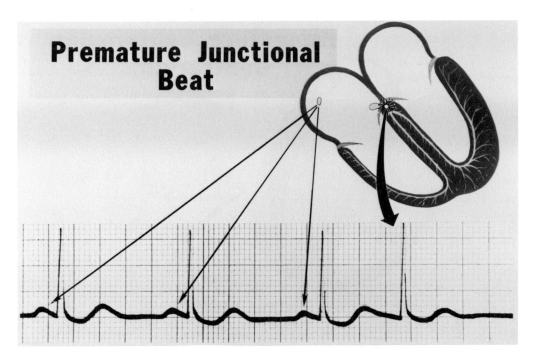

Premature Junctional Beat

A *Premature Junctional Beat* is produced by a sudden discharge from an ectopic focus in the AV Junction, so the impulse continues down the ventricular conduction system pathway.

A Premature Junctional Beat originates in an ectopic focus in the AV Junction which fires before the _____ begins a normal cycle.

SA Node

Therefore one usually notices a normal* appearing _____ which occurs very early and is generally not preceded by a P wave.

QRS

> NOTE: The AV Junctional ectopic focus can send an impulse upward to stimulate the atria from below (RETROGRADE CONDUCTION). When it occurs, this backwards atrial depolarization may create an *inverted* P wave which can appear just before or just after the QRS, or this peculiar *inverted* P wave may be mixed in with the QRS complex.

*The QRS complexes which originate (prematurely or with rapid rates) in an ectopic Junctional or atrial ectopic focus occasionally may appear slightly wider than the other QRS complexes.

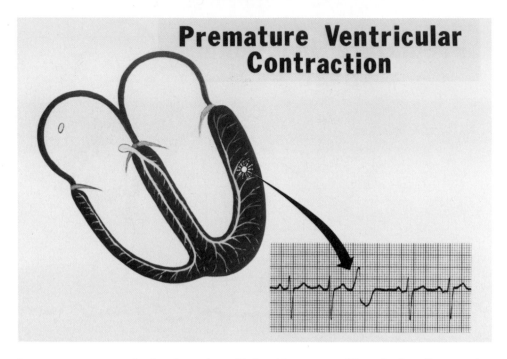

Premature Ventricular Contraction

A premature ventricular beat is called a *Premature Ventricular Contraction* (P.V.C.).* It originates suddenly in an ectopic focus in a ventricle producing a giant ventricular complex.

An ectopic focus may suddenly discharge an impulse from somewhere in one of the _____.

ventricles

This ventricular ectopic beat, like all other premature beats, occurs very early (before a _____ wave can begin a new cycle), and it is called a P.V.C.

P

The resultant Premature Ventricular Contraction, commonly known as a _____, is easily recognized on the electrocardiogram tracing by its enormous size.

P.V.C.

NOTE: P.V.C. denotes a ventricular "contraction." When you see a P.V.C., remember that there is a (premature) ventricular contraction and an associated pulse beat like that produced by a normal QRS, except it is earlier and usually weaker than normal.

*Some claim that P.V.C. stands for Premature Ventricular *Complex*, which more aptly describes what we see on the EKG tracing. Either is correct.

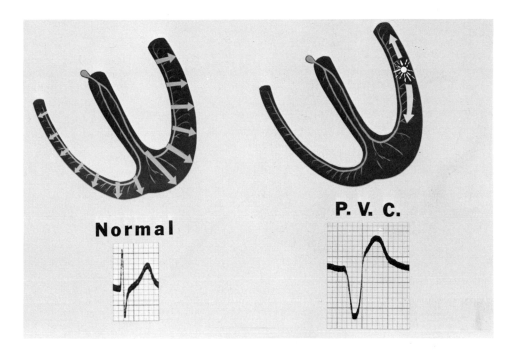

Normal

P. V. C.

Depolarization of the P.V.C. does not follow the usual ventricular conduction system pathway, therefore conduction is slow (very wide QRS).

The ventricular conduction system normally conducts the electrical stimulus of ventricular depolarization to all internal ventricular surfaces very rapidly, yielding a narrow QRS _____.

complex

However, depolarization of the P.V.C. originates in the myocardium (outside the ventricular conduction system), and the myocardial cells conduct the depolarization impulse very _____.

slowly

NOTE: The ventricular conduction system conducts impulses at a rate of 2–4 meters/second. Normal myocardium conducts electrical impulses at a rate of only one meter/second (without the aid of the ventricular conduction system). Therefore the nervous conduction system of the ventricles conducts electrical impulses 2 to 4 times faster than the muscle tissue (myocardium) can alone.

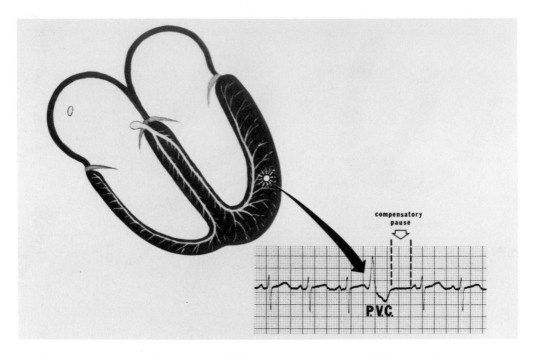

The P.V.C. is a much taller and deeper (as well as wider) complex than the normal QRS. There is a compensatory pause after the P.V.C.

There is a compensatory pause after a _____ during which the heart is electrically silent.   P.V.C.

NOTE: During normal ventricular conduction, the left and right ventricles depolarize simultaneously. As a result, depolarization going toward the left (left ventricle) is somewhat opposed by simultaneous depolarization going toward the right (right ventricle), and a relatively small (normal) QRS results. But a P.V.C. originates in one ventricle which depolarizes before the other. So the deflections of a P.V.C. are very tall and very deep (no simultaneous opposing depolarization from opposite sides) on the electrocardiogram. P.V.C.'s have greater deflections than normal QRS complexes.

NOTE: *Interpolated* P.V.C.'s are somehow sandwiched between the normal beats of a tracing, producing no compensatory pause and no disturbance in the normal regular rhythm.

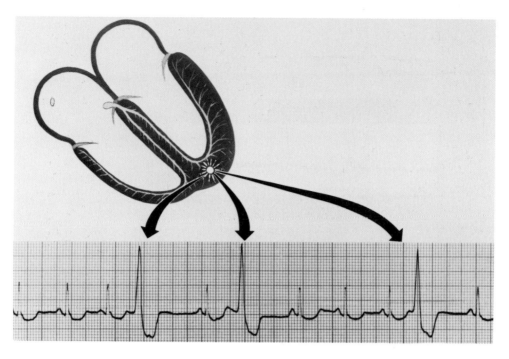

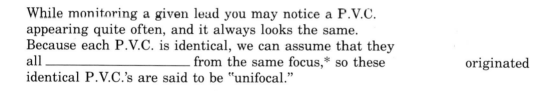

Numerous P.V.C.'s may originate from the same focus. Six or more P.V.C.'s per minute is considered pathological.

While monitoring a given lead you may notice a P.V.C. appearing quite often, and it always looks the same. Because each P.V.C. is identical, we can assume that they all _____ from the same focus,* so these   originated
identical P.V.C.'s are said to be "unifocal."

P.V.C.'s often indicate that the heart's own (coronary) blood supply is poor, so their appearance alerts us that something may be wrong. _____ P.V.C.'s per minute is   Six
pathological.

> NOTE: In cases where the coronary blood flow is adequate but the blood is poorly oxygenated (e.g., drowning, pulmonary pathology, tracheal obstruction, etc.), the heart recognizes poor oxygenation (and high CO_2) and ventricular ectopic foci will discharge frequently. Certain stimulants and medications may also spark P.V.C.'s.

*It is common to drop the adjective "ectopic" from ectopic focus.

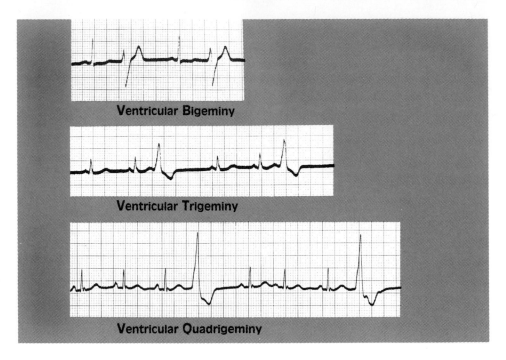

Ventricular Bigeminy

Ventricular Trigeminy

Ventricular Quadrigeminy

P.V.C.'s may become coupled with one or more normal cycles to produce Ventricular Bigeminy, Ventricular Trigeminy, etc.

P.V.C.'s occasionally become _____ with one or more normal cycles, and this pattern recurs over and over.

coupled

When a P.V.C. becomes coupled with a normal cycle, this is called Ventricular _____ as this pattern recurs with each normal cycle.

Bigeminy

If you were to see a P.V.C. apparently coupled with two normal cycles and the pattern repeats itself many times, one could call this runs of Ventricular

_____.

Trigeminy

Ventricular Parasystole

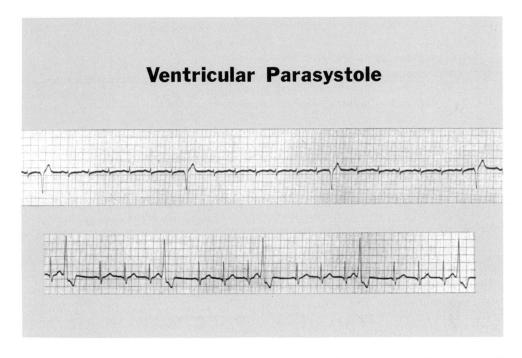

Ventricular Parasystole is a dual rhythm caused by two pacemakers, one of which is a ventricular ectopic focus (the other is usually the SA Node).

A ventricular ectopic pacemaker produces P.V.C.-like QRS complexes at a generally slow rate, but when associated with another (supraventricular) rhythm, this is known as ventricular _____.

parasystole

NOTE: The ventricular ectopic beats demonstrate a regular rhythmicity in parasystole, and because of a "protective" phenomenon, very few beats are dropped (non-conducted).

When you recognize P.V.C.'s that appear to be "coupled" to a long series of normal beats, you should suspect ventricular _____.

parasystole

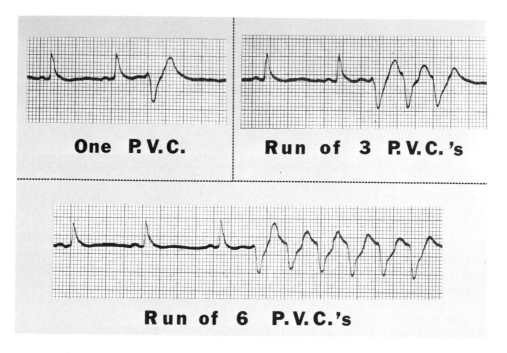

One P.V.C.   **Run of 3 P.V.C.'s**

Run of 6 P.V.C.'s

A single ventricular ectopic focus may fire once, or it may fire a series of successive impulses to produce a run of P.V.C.'s.

A single _____ ectopic focus may fire   ventricular
a series of discharges in rapid succession.

Runs of P.V.C.'s are considered more serious than occasional
single P.V.C.'s from a single _____, particularly with   focus
infarction patients.

NOTE: A run of three or more P.V.C.'s in rapid succession
is called a run of "Ventricular Tachycardia" (see the second
example in the above illustration), but we will go deeper
into this later.

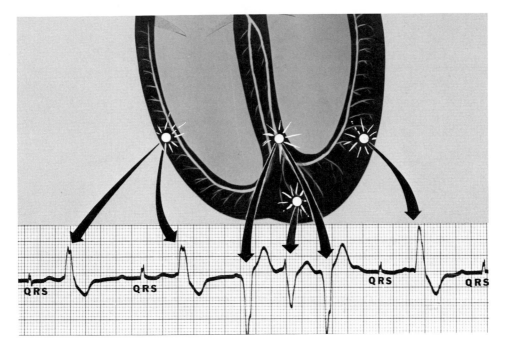

Multifocal P.V.C.'s are produced by multiple ventricular ectopic foci. Each focus produces an identical appearing P.V.C. every time it fires.

In a given lead P.V.C.'s originating from the _____ focus will appear the same.

same

NOTE: The appearance of numerous multifocal P.V.C.'s is indeed dangerous and requires rapid treatment. Because a single ventricular focus can take off and fire a series of rapid discharges causing dangerous arrhythmias (e.g., Ventricular Tachycardia), the appearance of numerous *multifocal* P.V.C.'s means that there are many foci discharging, and there is trouble ahead. The chance of developing a dangerous or even deadly arrhythmia (like Ventricular Fibrillation) under these circumstances is very much enhanced. With infarction patients this is a dire warning.

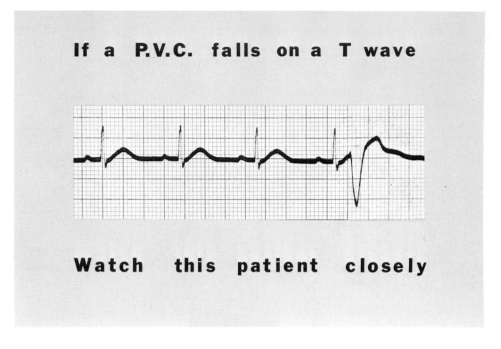

If a P.V.C. falls on a T wave

Watch this patient closely

If a P.V.C. falls on a T wave, it occurs during a vulnerable period and dangerous arrhythmias may result.

P.V.C.'s ordinarily occur just after the _____ wave of a normal cycle.

T

When a P.V.C. falls on a T wave of a normal cycle, it is catching the ventricles during a _____ period (this is called "R on T" phenomenon).

vulnerable

A P.V.C. which falls on a T wave may cause the _____ to beat rapidly.

ventricles

NOTE: Although considered a warning sign, *R on T* is often noted "after the fact", that is, when an EKG strip containing a spontaneous ventricular tachy-arrhythmia is examined closely, one may find that it was precipitated by this phenomenon.

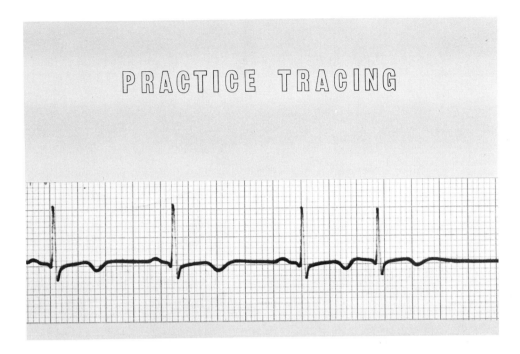

PRACTICE TRACING

The discerning eye of a Coronary Care Nurse detected a beat which appeared a little too early in an EKG strip taken from a patient's monitor.

By looking at the last QRS complex in the strip you discover that it is not preceded by a _____ wave.

P

The last QRS complex looks the same as the other QRS's, so we know that the last one followed the usual ventricular _____ system, therefore it did *not* originate in a ventricular focus.

conduction

The last ventricular depolarization (QRS complex) on this strip probably originated in the _____, and it is a premature beat.

AV Junction

NOTE: Please take a minute and run through the illustrations on page 101 through 113 to reinforce your understanding of these single beats which originate suddenly in an ectopic focus.

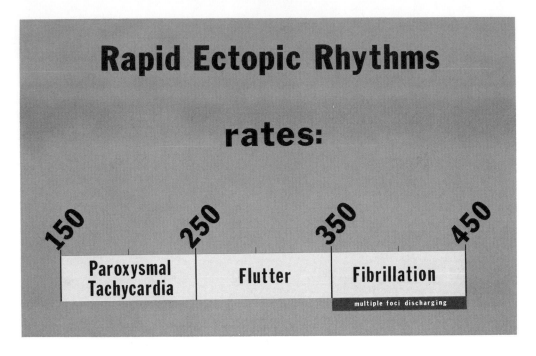

Rapid ectopic rhythms originate in an ectopic focus which is pacing rapidly. Sometimes more than one focus is involved.

The rates of the Rapid Ectopic Rhythms are:

Paroxysmal Tachycardia . . . . _____ to _____/min.   150 to 250
Flutter . . . . _____ to _____/min.   250 to 350
Fibrillation . . . . _____ to _____/min.   350 to 450

> NOTE: Rapid ectopic rhythms are easily recognized by rate alone, but the diagnosis involves identification of the location of the ectopic focus that is responsible. A basic understanding* of normal conduction within the heart, as well as an insight into the location and function of these foci, is the key to a practical knowledge of these *tachy-arrhythmias.*

*"Understanding is a kind of ecstasy." Carl Sagan (from *Broca's Brain*).

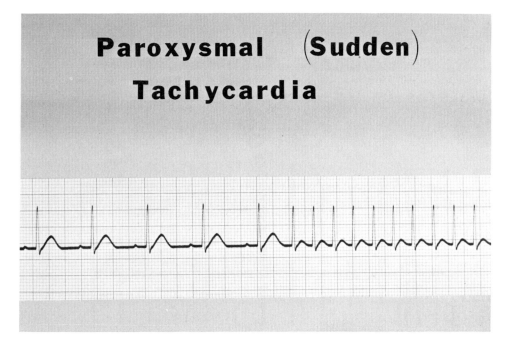

Paroxysmal (Sudden) Tachycardia

Paroxysmal Tachycardia means "sudden," "rapid heart rate" (150 to 250 per minute) which originates in an ectopic focus.

_____ means a rapid heart rate.   Tachycardia

Paroxysmal means _____.   sudden

Paroxysmal Tachycardia usually arises spontaneously from
an ectopic focus which fires impulses in _____   rapid
succession at the rate of 150 to 250 per minute.

> NOTE: The normal pacemaker, the SA Node, may
> gradually increase the heart rate in certain conditions.
> This is called a "Sinus" Tachycardia since it originates in
> the SA Node (Sinus Node), and it is often due to
> excitement, exercise, stimulating drugs, shock, etc. Sinus
> Tachycardia is NOT a Paroxysmal Tachycardia.

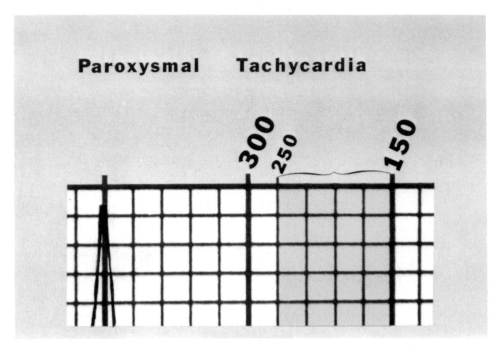

The rate range of the paroxysmal tachycardias is 150–250/minute, so they are easy to recognize. Identifying the location of the rapidly pacing focus gives us the diagnosis.

When calculating rate, we find an R wave which peaks on a heavy black line. The next three heavy black lines are called "300, 150, _____".

100

The fine line just to the right of the line named "300" is 250. Therefore, if an R wave falls on the first heavy black line (above illustration), the next R wave will fall within the shaded area during a paroxysmal _____.

tachycardia

Now you should be able to recognize a paroxysmal tachycardia by noting the rate range of _____ to 250. Let's go on to identify the location of the ectopic focus (in the atria, AV Junction, or ventricles) which is rapidly pacing, and this will make our diagnosis.

150

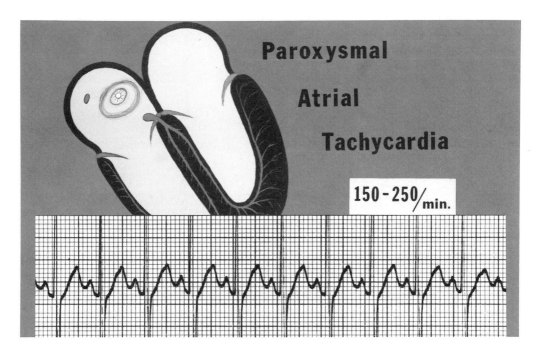

Paroxysmal Atrial Tachycardia is caused by the sudden, rapid firing of an ectopic atrial pacemaker.

Paroxysmal Atrial Tachycardia is a _____, rapid heart rate originating from an ectopic focus in one of the atria. The rate is usually 150 to 250/minute.

sudden

Because the focus is ectopic, the P waves in P.A.T. usually do not look like the other P waves (before the tachycardia) in the same _____.

lead

Each ectopic impulse stimulates the _____ and then is conducted down the normal ventricular conduction system pathway, yielding normal appearing P-QRS-T cycles.

atria

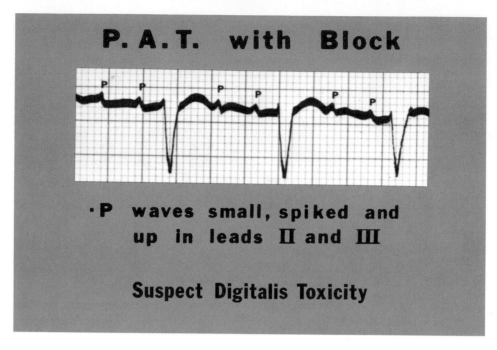

In *Paroxysmal Atrial Tachycardia with block* there is more than one P wave spike for every QRS response. This often signifies digitalis toxicity.

NOTE: This is basically a (paroxysmal) atrial tachycardia originating in an atrial ectopic focus.

P.A.T. with block is recognized by the fact that each of the individual P wave spikes does not have a QRS response, i.e., every-other atrial impulse is blocked and does not get through the _____.   AV Node

So we may see two (or more) spiked "P waves" for each _____, but there is still an atrial tachycardia.   QRS

P.A.T. with block is often an indication of digitalis _____, particularly when the serum potassium   toxicity
is low, so giving potassium is usually helpful.

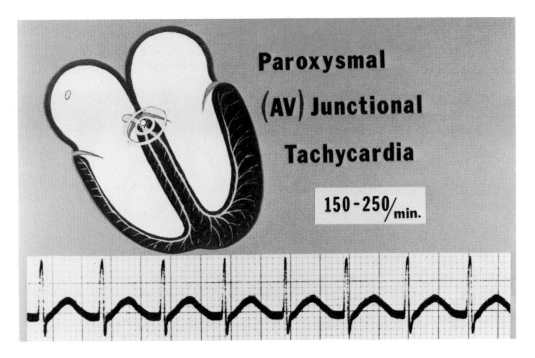

Paroxysmal Junctional Tachycardia is caused by the sudden, rapid pacing of an ectopic focus in the AV Junction.

Paroxysmal Junctional Tachycardia is due to a rapid pace (150–250) set by an ectopic focus in the

_____.   AV Junction

> NOTE: Ectopic foci in the AV Junction can stimulate the atria from below by retrograde conduction. This may produce *inverted* P waves immediately before or just after each QRS complex in the tachycardia. Also, the QRS complexes may appear slightly wider than normal in P.J.T. because of aberrant ventricular conduction.

> NOTE: A putative "AV Nodal Re-entry Tachycardia" allegedly occurs when a wave of current passes retrograde from the AV Node to adjacent atrial tissue and back through the AV Node as a repeating circular ("circus") wave phenomenon. Each circular pass stimulates the ventricles then the atria at a tachycardia rate.

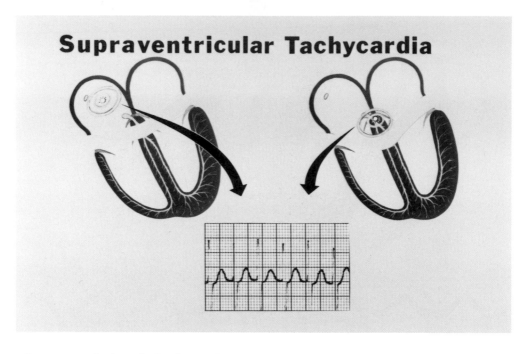

Supraventricular Tachycardia

Paroxysmal Atrial Tachycardia and Paroxysmal Junctional Tachycardia may be considered as originating above the ventricles and are known as paroxysmal "Supraventricular Tachycardia."

Paroxysmal Atrial Tachycardia and Paroxysmal Junctional Tachycardia both originate* above the ventricles and are generally known as (paroxysmal)

_____ Tachycardia.   Supraventricular

NOTE: Paroxysmal Atrial Tachycardia may occur at such a rapid rate that the P waves run into the preceding T waves and appear like one wave. This makes the differentiation of these two tachycardias very difficult; however, because they are both treated in the same manner, differentiation of P.A.T. and P.J.T. is not essential. So if we cannot make a distinction between the two, we can just say "Supraventricular Tachycardia."

NOTE: Any beat of atrial or Junctional ectopic origin may be called "supraventricular," and if premature or with a tachycardia rate, a slightly widened QRS complex may result from aberrant ventricular conduction.

*Although illustrations commonly depict the His Bundle (and the AV Junction) within the interventricular septum, it is really oriented horizontally along the *top* of the septum and is therefore truly SUPRAventricular.

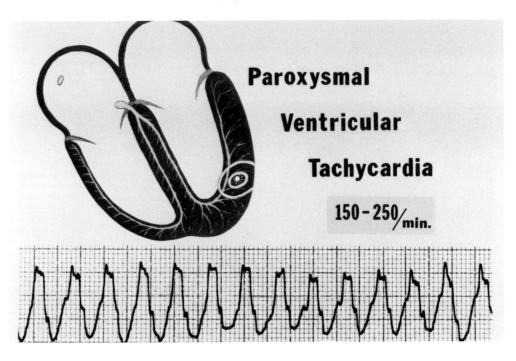

Paroxysmal Ventricular Tachycardia is produced by a rapidly discharging ventricular ectopic focus. It has a characteristic pattern with enormous P.V.C.-like ventricular complexes.

Paroxysmal Ventricular Tachycardia originates suddenly in an ectopic focus in one of the _____,   ventricles
producing a (ventricular) rate of 150–250.

Sudden runs of Ventricular Tachycardia* appear like a rapid series or _____ of P.V.C.'s (which in reality it is).   run

NOTE: Although the atria still depolarize regularly at their own inherent rate, distinct P waves are only occasionally seen. This independent atrial and ventricular pacing is known as *AV dissociation* (or simply "dissociation").

*The "Paroxysmal" is commonly left off.

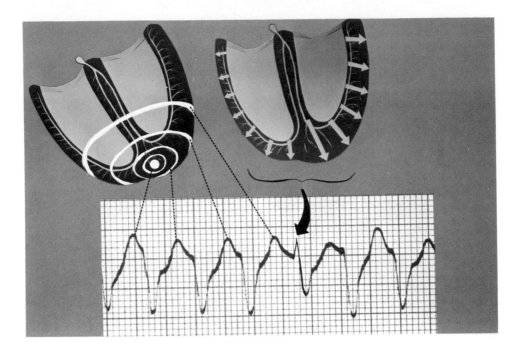
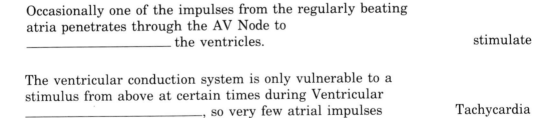

An occasional atrial impulse may penetrate through the AV Node from above to stimulate a normal appearing ventricular complex during Ventricular Tachycardia.

Occasionally one of the impulses from the regularly beating atria penetrates through the AV Node to
_____ the ventricles.

stimulate

The ventricular conduction system is only vulnerable to a stimulus from above at certain times during Ventricular _____, so very few atrial impulses penetrate through the AV Node with the proper timing to stimulate the ventricles.

Tachycardia

> NOTE: When the ventricular conduction system occasionally is stimulated by an atrial depolarization from above (during Ventricular Tachycardia), the impulse can follow the normal ventricular conduction system pathway producing a nearly normal-looking portion of a QRS which fuses with a P.V.C.-type complex (already progressing from the ectopic focus), creating a "Fusion Beat." Rarely, the impulse from above will be carried to completion to capture a normal QRS, creating a "Capture Beat." The presence of "captures" or "fusions" confirms our diagnosis of Ventricular Tachycardia.

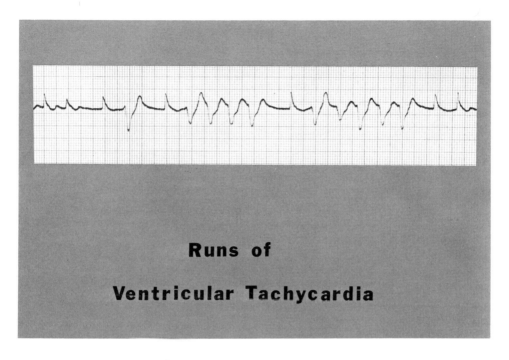

Runs of

Ventricular Tachycardia

Runs of (Paroxysmal) Ventricular Tachycardia may signify coronary artery disease or hypoxia.

Ventricular Tachycardia appears like a run of
_____.   P.V.C.'s

This is a pathological condition and usually signifies
coronary _____ disease or poor oxygenation of the   artery
heart (other causes).

> NOTE: This rapid ventricular rate originates from a
> ventricular ectopic focus, and the rate is really too fast for
> the heart to function effectively, so it should be treated
> quickly, particularly in the patient with an infarction.
> There is an unusual form of ventricular tachycardia which
> is illustrated on page 268.

> CAUTION: Rapid Junctional or rapid atrial
> (supraventricular) rhythms may produce widened QRS's
> (because of aberrant ventricular conduction) which can
> mimic Ventricular Tachycardia.

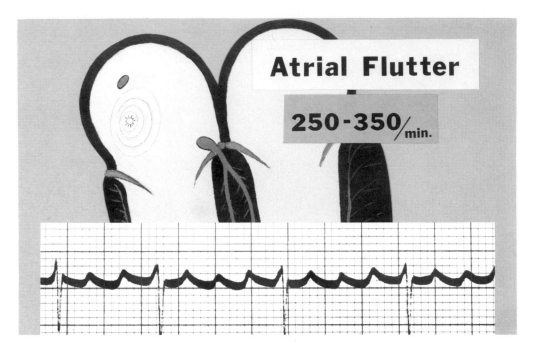

Atrial Flutter originates in an atrial ectopic focus. P waves occur in rapid succession and each is identical to the next.

In atrial flutter an ectopic focus in the atria fires at a rate of 250–350 to produce a rapid succession of _____ depolarizations.

atrial

> NOTE: The diagnosis of Atrial Flutter is most often made on the basis of appearance rather than rate.

Because there is only one ectopic _____ discharging, each "P wave" looks identical to all the others. The atrial depolarizations originate ectopically so they are not really P waves, and therefore they are often called flutter waves.

focus

It is only the occasional atrial stimulus which will penetrate through the AV Node, so there are a few flutter waves in series before a _____ response is seen.

QRS

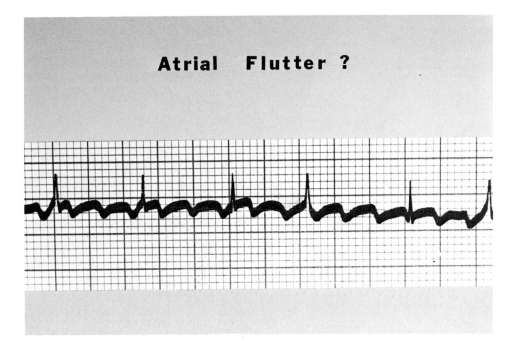

Atrial Flutter ?

This tracing looks somewhat like atrial flutter, but to make it more classical you have to turn it upside down.

When in doubt about atrial flutter, inverting the _____ may be very helpful.   tracing

> NOTE: Atrial flutter is characterized by a series of identical "P waves" in rapid succession or back-to-back flutter waves. Because the waves are identical, they are described as having the appearance of the teeth of a saw or "saw tooth" baseline. It is important to note that the waves fall in rapid succession, and there is usually no flat baseline between them. Turn back to P.A.T. with block and make sure you understand the difference.

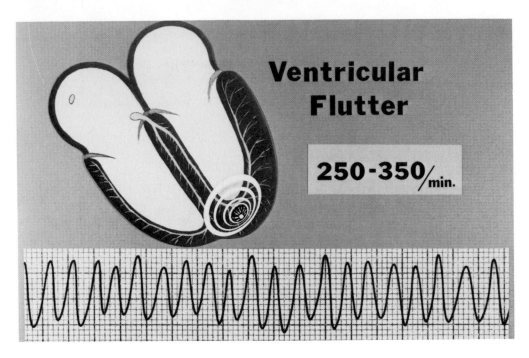

Ventricular Flutter is produced by a single ventricular ectopic focus firing at the extremely rapid rate of 250 to 350/min. Notice the smooth sine wave appearance.

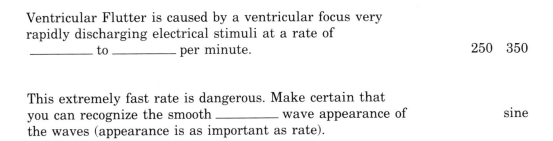

Ventricular Flutter is caused by a ventricular focus very rapidly discharging electrical stimuli at a rate of
_____ to _____ per minute.

250   350

This extremely fast rate is dangerous. Make certain that you can recognize the smooth _____ wave appearance of the waves (appearance is as important as rate).

sine

NOTE: Ventricular Flutter deteriorates into deadly arrhythmias.

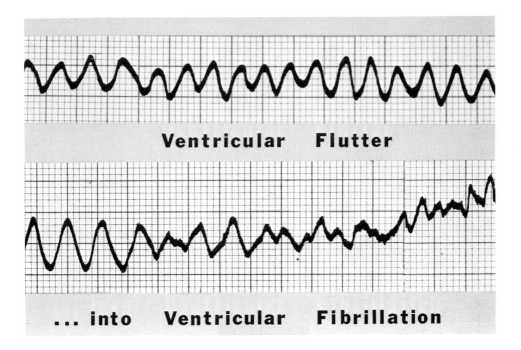

Ventricular Flutter

... into Ventricular Fibrillation

True Ventricular Flutter almost invariably becomes Ventricular Fibrillation requiring cardio-pulmonary resuscitation and defibrillation.

NOTE: During Ventricular Flutter the ventricles are contracting at an incredible rate. The above tracings show Ventricular Flutter at a rate of about 300 per minute, or 5 contractions per second. Blood is a viscous fluid, and the ventricles cannot be filled at a rate of 5 times per second, so there is virtually no ventricular filling. For this reason there is no effective cardiac output. The coronary arteries are not receiving blood at this rate, and the heart itself has no blood supply. Ventricular Fibrillation results as the many ventricular ectopic foci desperately try to compensate.

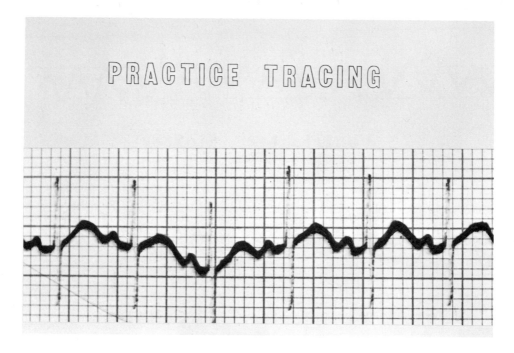

PRACTICE TRACING

A monitored patient became very concerned about a *sudden* pounding in his chest.

By the history and the rate (which you quickly determined by inspection), you identify this rhythm as a paroxysmal tachy-_____. Now you must identify the causative ectopic focus.

cardia

Because this paroxysmal tachycardia has narrow, normal looking QRS's, it could *not* have originated in a _____ ectopic focus, so it must be some type of supraventricular tachycardia.

ventricular

There appear to be P waves present, so we are probably dealing with an _____ ectopic focus. Ah, but now you remember that a Junctional focus may occasionally produce a P wave just before or after the QRS; however, a Junctional focus produces *inverted* P waves!

atrial

NOTE: This is Paroxysmal Atrial Tachycardia, and because all P waves are conducted to produce a QRS response, it could not be P.A.T. with block. Please take a moment to review the illustrations on pages 114 through 128.

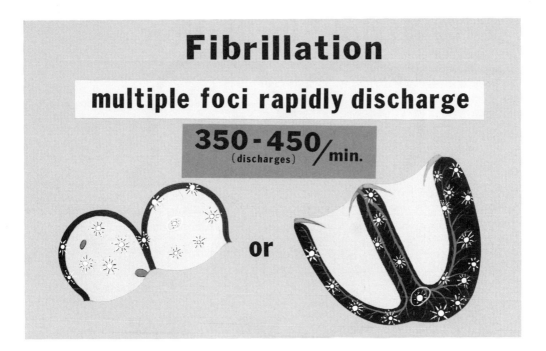

Fibrillation

multiple foci rapidly discharge

350-450/min.
(discharges)

or

Fibrillation is an erratic rhythm caused by continuous, rapid-rate discharges from numerous ectopic foci of the same level (either in the atria or in the ventricles).

NOTE: Fibrillation is caused by rapid discharges from numerous ectopic foci in the atria (Atrial Fibrillation), or due to numerous foci of the ventricles rapidly discharging (Ventricular Fibrillation). The result is so erratic and uncoordinated that distinct, complete waves are not distinguishable, and therefore rates are difficult to determine. The involved chambers merely twitch rapidly.

NOTE: The rate, 350 to 450 per minute, is not a true rate, since many of the multiple foci may discharge simultaneously. Both the number and the tachy-rate of individual foci is conjectural. The rate range is more relative and hypothetical than real.

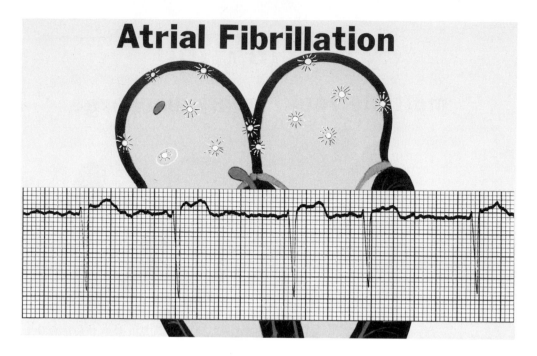

Atrial Fibrillation

Atrial Fibrillation is caused by *many* atrial ectopic foci firing at rapid rates causing an exceedingly rapid, erratic atrial rhythm (atrial "rate" 350 to 450/min).

Atrial _____ occurs when many ecoptic foci in the atria fire rapidly, producing an excessively rapid series of tiny erratic spikes on EKG (no P waves).

Fibrillation

NOTE: Only a small portion of the atria is depolarized by any one ectopic impulse, and because so many ectopic foci are rapidly firing, no one discharge is carried far.

NOTE: With a normal rhythm the SA Node sends out an impulse which spreads through the atria like an enlarging circular wave caused by throwing a pebble in a still pool of water. The multiple erratic depolarizations of atrial fibrillation are analogous to rain falling into the same pool.

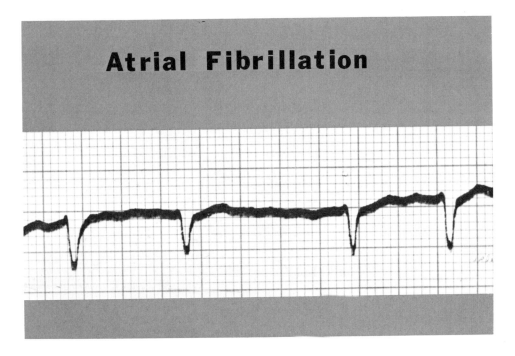

Atrial Fibrillation

Atrial Fibrillation often appears only as an irregular baseline without P waves. The QRS response is *not* regular and may be rapid or slow.

Atrial Fibrillation may cause such small, erratic spikes that it appears as an irregular baseline without visible _____ waves or tiny spikes.

P

The AV Node is irregularly stimulated during atrial fibrillation, so the ventricular _____ is likewise generally irregular. (Therefore expect an irregular pulse.)

response

NOTE: The ventricular rate depends on the AV Node's responsiveness to multiple small stimuli, so the ventricular rate may be rapid or relatively slow, but *it is always irregular.* You must determine and document the general (average) ventricular rate (QRS's per 6-sec. strip times 10).

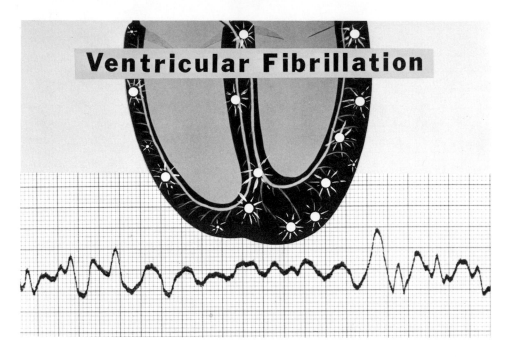

Ventricular Fibrillation is caused by rapid-rate discharges from *many* ventricular ectopic foci producing an erratic, rapid twitching of the ventricles (ventricular "rate" 350 to 450/min).

_____ Fibrillation originates in numerous ventricular ectopic foci each of which fires at a rapid rate.

Ventricular

Because there are so many ventricular ectopic _____ firing at once, each of which only depolarizes a small area of ventricle, this results in a rapid, erratic twitching of the ventricles.

foci

This erratic twitching is often called a "bag of worms" for this is the way the ventricles really appear. There is no effective _____ pumping, and the tracing of ventricular fibrillation is characteristically erratic.

cardiac

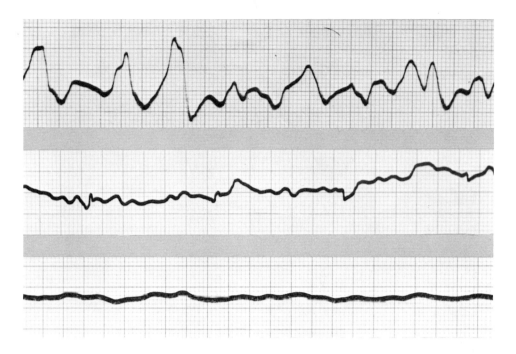

Ventricular Fibrillation is easily recognized by its totally erratic appearance.

Ventricular Fibrillation is easily recognized by the totally
_____ appearance on the tracing, and even with   erratic
large deflections there are no identifiable waves.

There is no predictable pattern of _____   Ventricular
Fibrillation. As you can see, it appears different at every
moment, but it is so erratic that it is difficult to miss.

If you *do* recognize any repetition of pattern or regularity of
deflections, you probably are not dealing with Ventricular
_____.   Fibrillation

NOTE: These three strips are a continuous tracing of the
same patient's dying heart. Notice how the amplitude of
the deflections becomes less as the heart dies.

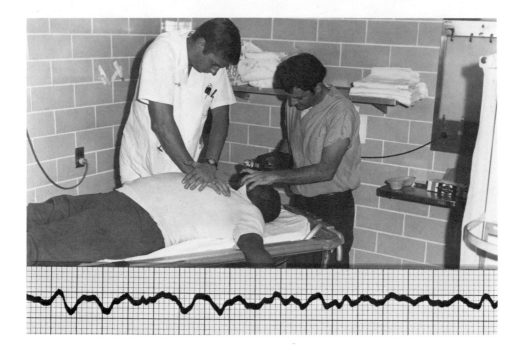

In Ventricular Fibrillation there is no pumping action of the heart (*Cardiac Arrest*); this is a dire emergency!

Ventricular Fibrillation is a type of Cardiac Arrest. There is no effective cardiac output, because the ventricles are only twitching erratically, and there is no ventricular
_____—i.e., no circulation.   pumping

NOTE: There are two other types of Cardiac Arrest: *Standstill* ("Asystole") occurs when there is no detectable cardiac activity, producing only flat baseline on EKG. *Electro-Mechanical Dissociation* (E.M.D.) is present when a dying heart produces weak EKG signs of electrical activity, but the heart is too moribund to respond mechanically.

NOTE: Cardiac Arrest is an emergency situation which requires immediate care (external cardiac massage and artificial respiration) known as Cardio-Pulmonary Resuscitation. The technique of C.P.R. was originally taught only to hospital and ambulance personnel, but it is now imperative that every living person be adept at this technique. In this way immediate resuscitation may be rendered to people suddenly stricken with Ventricular Fibrillation (or other type of Cardiac Arrest) in any locale or situation.

NOTE: Let's quickly review the illustrations on pages 129 to 134.

Heart Blocks

Sinus Block

AV Block

Bundle Branch Block

Hemiblock   (begins page 245)

Heart Blocks* can occur in the SA Node, AV Node, or in the larger sections of the ventricular conduction system.

Heart Blocks may occur in any of these areas: the SA Node, the AV Node, the His Bundle, in the _____ Branches, or in one of the two divisions of the Left Bundle Branch (Hemiblock).

Bundle

_____ Blocks are electrical blocks which retard (or prevent) the passage of electrical (depolarization) stimuli.

Heart

NOTE: When examining the rhythm on a tracing, you must ALWAYS check for *all* varieties of Heart Blocks, because the same patient may have more than one type of block.

*"Heart Blocks" is a colloquial term which is more commonly referred to simply as "Blocks" in most medical circles.

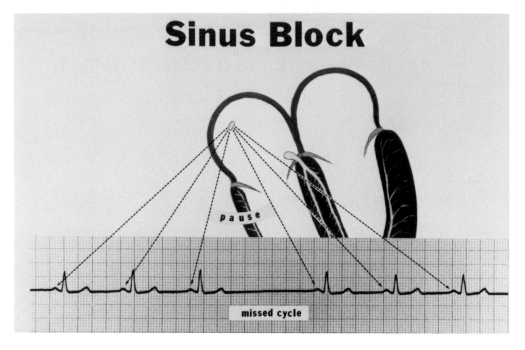

Sinus Block

pause

missed cycle

An unhealthy Sinus Node (SA Node) may temporarily fail to pace for at least one cycle ("Sinus Block"), but then it resumes pacing.

With Sinus Block (also called "SA Node Block" or simply "SA Block") an unhealthy SA Node* stops its pacing activity for at least one complete _____.   cycle

After the pause pacing resumes at the same rate (and timing) as prior to the block, as the _____ Node resumes   SA
pacing activity. However, the pause may evoke an *escape beat* from an impatient ectopic focus before SA Node pacing can resume.

> NOTE: The P waves before and after the block are identical because the same SA Node pacemaker is functioning before and after the pause (i.e., all P waves originate in the SA Node). But a long pause may elicit an "escape" beat from an ectopic focus before the SA Node resumes pacing.

*Some experts claim that the SA Node propagates a stimulus, but that it is blocked from exiting the Node. This is referred to as "Sinus Exit Block."

AV BLOCK

1° (first degree) AV Block

2° (second degree) AV Block

3° (third degree) AV Block

Atrio-Ventricular (AV) *Block*, when minimal, delays the impulse (from the atria) within the AV Node, making a longer-than-normal pause before stimulating the ventricles. More serious AV Blocks may totally stop some (or all) atrial stimuli from reaching the ventricles.

In its most innocuous form an AV _____ delays the atrial impulse before it continues on to be conducted to the ventricular myocardium.

Block

> NOTE: You will recall that there is a brief pause between atrial depolarization and ventricular stimulation. This pause between the P wave and QRS complex is lengthened* on the EKG tracing when a minor AV Block is present. More serious AV Blocks will completely block some (or all) impulses from reaching the ventricles (on EKG a P wave with no QRS response).

> NOTE: The three varieties of AV Block are:
>   *first degree* (1°) *AV Block*
>   *second degree* (2°) *AV Block*
>   *third degree* (3°) *AV Block*
> I will use their alternate designations (in parentheses) so that you will become familiar with both ways of expressing each block, since both designations are common in current literature.

*This lengthening is manifested as a prolonged P-R interval (see next page).

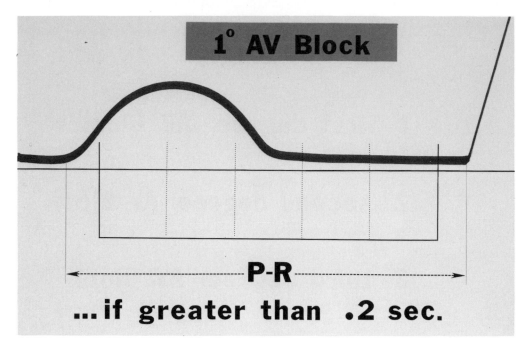

1° AV Block

P-R

...if greater than .2 sec.

The delay of *first degree (1°) AV Block* prolongs the P-R interval more than one large square (.2 sec.) on EKG.

The delay caused by 1° AV Block prolongs the P-R
_____.   interval

> NOTE: Although "segments" are portions of baseline, an "interval" contains at least one wave. So the P-R interval includes the P wave and the baseline that follows it up to the point where the QRS complex begins. The P-R interval is measured from the beginning of the P wave to the beginning of the QRS complex.

The P-R interval normally should measure less than one
large square or less than ____ second.   .2
                                                                        (2/10)

> NOTE: You must observe the P-R intervals on every EKG, for if *any* P-R interval is longer than one large square, some kind of AV Block is present.

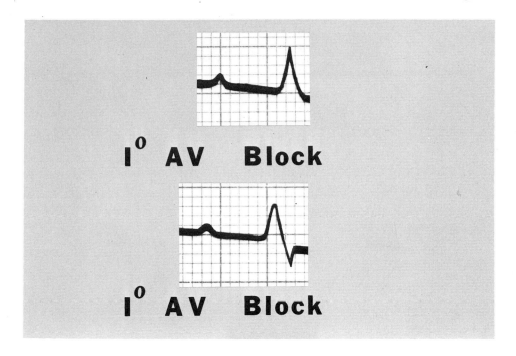

A *first degree AV Block* is characterized by a P-R interval greater than .2 sec. (one large square). The amount of P-R prolongation is consistent with each cycle.

Once you recognize a prolonged P-R _____, you should determine the type of AV Block which is present.

interval

Some type of AV Block is present if any _____ interval is longer than .2 second.

P-R

A _____ AV Block is present when the P-QRS-T sequence is normal, but the P-R interval is prolonged *the same amount in every cycle.*

first degree
(1°)

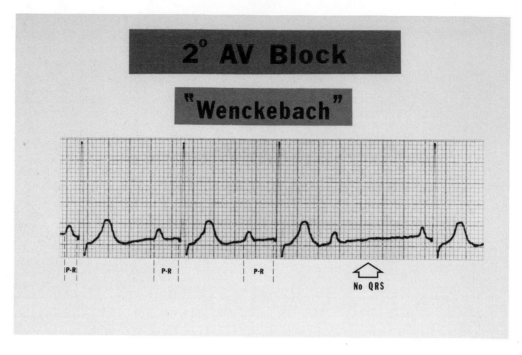

The *Wenckebach phenomenon* is a *second degree AV Block* in which the P-R interval becomes progressively longer until the AV Node is not penetrated (no QRS).

The Wenckebach phenomenon (pronounced Winky-bok) occurs when the AV Block prolongs the P-R _____ progressively with each succeeding cycle.

interval

The P-R interval becomes gradually longer from cycle to cycle until the final P wave does not elicit a _____ response.

QRS

The P wave and QRS complex get farther apart in successive cycles. The last P _____ stands alone. This series repeats.

wave

> NOTE: Wenckebach phenomenon is a type of 2° AV Block. This is also referred to as *Type I*. Because the PR lengthening is gradual, you must discipline yourself to routinely scan series of cycles for same in each EKG you examine.

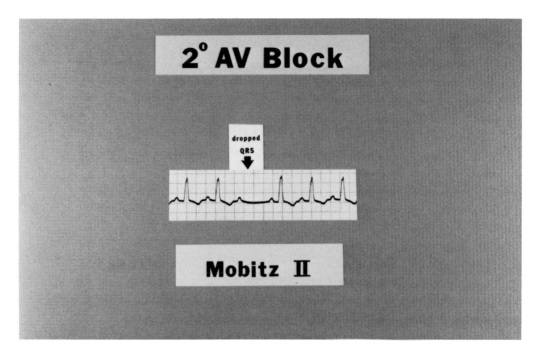

Occasionally, without lengthening the P-R interval, a QRS is dropped. This is *Mobitz II**, a type of *second degree AV Block*.

Mobitz II is noted when an occasional ventricular depolarization (QRS) is not conducted ("dropped") after a normal P wave, and there are generally normal, uniform P-R intervals in the _____ and following cycles.

preceding
(previous)

> NOTE: Mobitz II block often heralds more serious conduction problems with progressively more involved blocking of ventricular conduction.

An occasional dropped QRS complex generally indicates a _____ 2° AV Block.

Mobitz II

> NOTE: Careful! Do not confuse this with Sinus Block in which the entire P-QRS-T cycle is missing.

*This is a forshortened, colloquialized form of the proper nomenclature, "Mobitz, Type II".

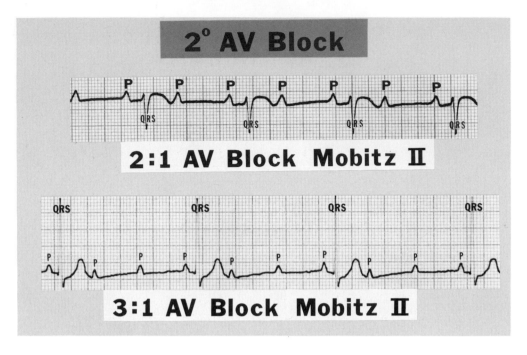

A *Mobitz II (second degree) AV Block* may cause every-other QRS to be blocked causing a two (P waves) to one (QRS) pattern to emerge.

NOTE: Return to the illustration on the previous page and visualize how a repetition of that block pattern becomes the upper tracing on this page (voila!).

A Mobitz II 2° AV Block may appear as two P waves (at a normal rate) to one QRS response, often referred to as 2:1 AV _____.   Block

This 2:1 AV Block (Mobitz II) really means every-other _____ complex is dropped, and it makes a nice tracing   QRS
for a book cover (you might glance at this book's cover).

Sometimes a Mobitz II (second degree) AV Block can require 3 atrial depolarizations (normal rate) to elicit a single _____ response; this is written 3:1 AV   ventricular
Block, and it describes the mechanism of conduction. Poor conduction ratios (e.g., 3:1, 4:1, etc.) relate to *increased severity* of the block and are sometimes called "advanced" Mobitz II AV Block.

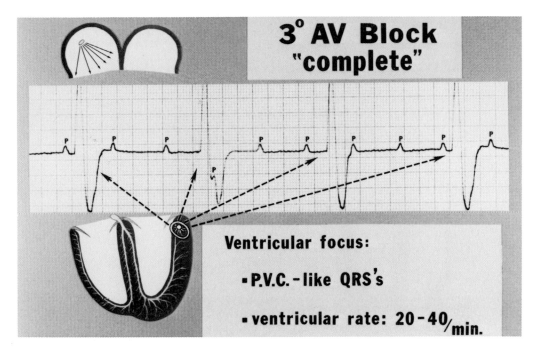

Third degree ("complete") *AV Block* occurs when none of the atrial impulses can get to the ventricles (no ventricular response). The ventricles must be paced independently.

In 3° (third degree) AV Block none of the atrial depolarizations penetrate through to the ventricles. This is a "_____ " AV Block.   complete

> NOTE: In 3° block, the block is "complete," that is, no atrial impulses get through to the ventricles. As a result, the ventricles (or AV Junction) call into action an ectopic (focus) pacemaker. In Complete Block there is an atrial rate and an independent ventricular rate. If the QRS's appear generally normal, the rhythm is said to be "idiojunctional" (Junctional pacemaker); but if the ventricular complexes are P.V.C.-like, (see illustration), then the rhythm is called "idioventricular" (ventricular pacemaker). The location of the ectopic focus (pacemaker) is sometimes assumed by the ventricular rate, i.e., ventricular rate of 40 to 60—Junctional ectopic pacemaker; ventricular rate of 20–40 is a ventricular ectopic pacemaker (illustration).

One will find a certain atrial (P wave) rate and an independent, usually slower, _____   ventricular
rate in third degree AV Block. This is a form of AV Dissociation.

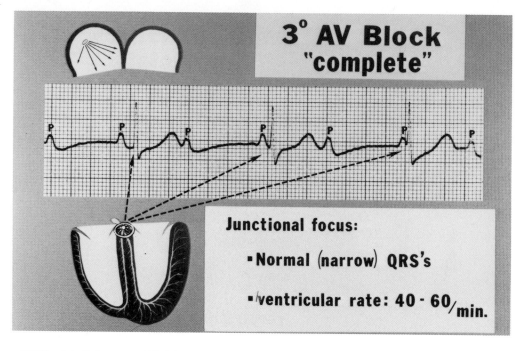

With third degree AV Block an ectopic focus in the unstimulated ventricles begins pacing at its own slow (20–40/min.) inherent rate, or an ectopic Junctional focus (illustration) may pace at its inherent rate of 40 to 60 per minute.

NOTE: The ectopic focus is identified by ventricular rate and QRS morphology.

Very slow rates are calculated by taking the cycles per six second strip and multiplying by _____.

ten

In the illustration a _____ ectopic focus (pacemaker) is setting the ventricular rate. Notice the normal, independent atrial rate (AV Dissociation).

Junctional

NOTE: In 3° AV Block the pulse (ventricular rate) may be so slow that the blood flow to the brain is diminished. As a result, a person with *complete* AV Block may lose consciousness and need to have his airway maintained. This is Stokes-Adams Syndrome.*

*Patients with Stokes-Adams Syndrome require the (surgical) implantation of an artificial pacemaker, however, a temporary non-invasive pacemaker (see page 274) is therapeutic.

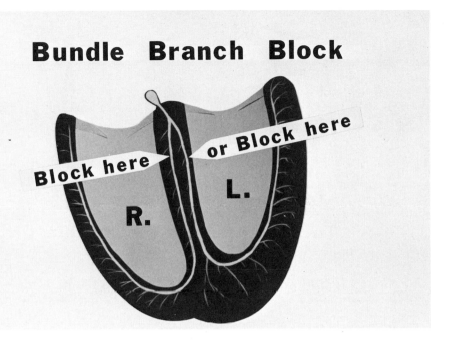

Bundle Branch Block

Bundle Branch Block is caused by a block (of depolarization) in the Right or in the Left Bundle Branch.

Normally the Right Bundle Branch quickly transmits the stimulus of depolarization to the _____ ventricle, and the Left Bundle Branch does the same to the left ventricle. This depolarization stimulus is transmitted to both ventricles at the same time (i.e., simultaneously).

right

A block to either of the Bundle Branches creates a delay of the _____ impulse to that side.

electrical
(depolarization)

Ordinarily both ventricles are _____ simultaneously.

depolarized
(or stimulated)

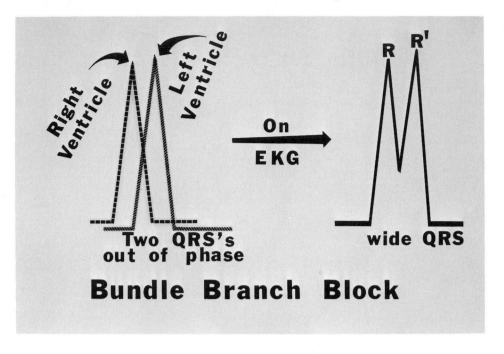

Bundle Branch Block

Therefore, in Bundle Branch Block one ventricle depolarizes slightly later than the other, causing two "joined QRS's."

When a Bundle Branch Block is present, either the left or the right _____ may depolarize late,   **ventricle** depending on which side is blocked.

> NOTE: The individual depolarization of the right ventricle and depolarization of the left ventricle are still of normal duration. Because the ventricles do not fire simultaneously, it produces the "widened QRS" appearance that we see on EKG. The two out-of-sync QRS's are superimposed on one-another, and the machine records it as a widened QRS.

Because the "widened QRS" represents the nonsimultaneous depolarization of both ventricles, one can usually see two R _____ named in order: R and R'. (R' represents the   **waves** late firing ventricle.)

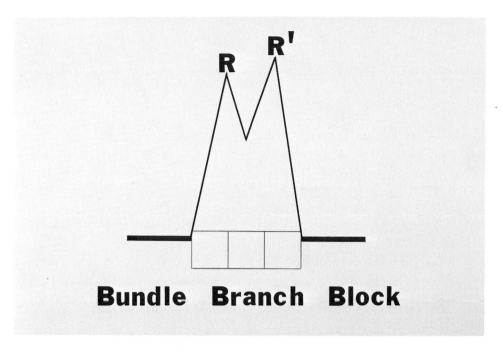

Bundle Branch Block

In Bundle Branch Block the QRS is 3 small squares wide (.12 sec.) or greater, and two R waves (R and R′) are seen.

The diagnosis of Bundle Branch Block is made mainly by the widened _____ (12/100 second or more).

QRS

In order to make the diagnosis of Bundle Branch Block, the QRS complex should be at least _____ small squares wide (or .12 sec.). Make certain that you check the width of the QRS routinely on every EKG that you read.

three

> NOTE: The needle which records the EKG tracing moves rapidly enough to record accurately most of the heart's electrical activity. However, with great deflections the needle lags a bit mechanically. The QRS deflections in the chest leads may be so great that the needle (inaccurately) records a QRS of a longer duration than it is in reality. For this reason it is often wise to routinely check the limb leads for QRS width.

> NOTE: If a patient with a Bundle Branch Block develops a supraventricular tachycardia, the rapid succession of widened QRS's may imitate Ventricular Tachycardia. Be careful!

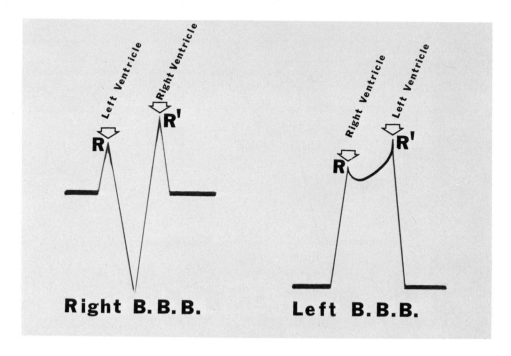

In Left Bundle Branch Block the left ventricle depolarizes late; in Right Bundle Branch Block the right ventricle depolarizes late.

In Bundle Branch Block you first notice a widened
_____. Then you should be able to find the R,R'
configuration in the chest leads.   QRS

In Right Bundle Branch Block the _____ ventricle   left
depolarizes punctually, so the R' represents delayed activity
from the right ventricle.

In Left Bundle Branch Block the left ventricular impulse is
delayed, so the right _____ depolarizes first   ventricle
and is followed by the delayed depolarization of the left
ventricle (R').

NOTE: Bundle Branch Block infers a block of one branch.
Depolarization progresses very slowly through the blocked
region of the blocked bundle branch and produces a
(delayed) stimulus to that branch below the block (thus the
delay).

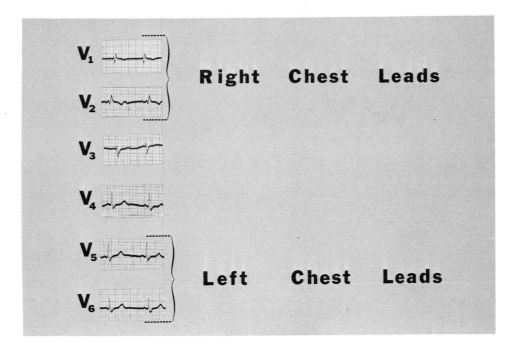

If there is a Bundle Branch Block, look at leads V_1 and V_2 (right chest leads) and leads V_5 and V_6 (left chest leads) for the R,R′.

When the QRS complex is wide enough to make the diagnosis of Bundle Branch Block, one immediately checks the right and left chest _____ for the R,R′.

leads

> NOTE: During ventricular depolarization and just afterward (up to the peak of the T wave), any additional stimulus cannot depolarize the ventricles, that is, they are *refractory* to any stimulus. Occasionally this refractory period varies between the two ventricles, so at a certain rapid (critical) rate or after early (premature) supraventricular beats, one ventricle begins to depolarize, but there may be a slight delay before the other ventricle can respond. This unusual type of ventricular conduction (called "aberrant conduction") may imitate a classical Bundle Branch Block because it also widens the QRS.

The right chest leads are V_1 and _____.

V_2

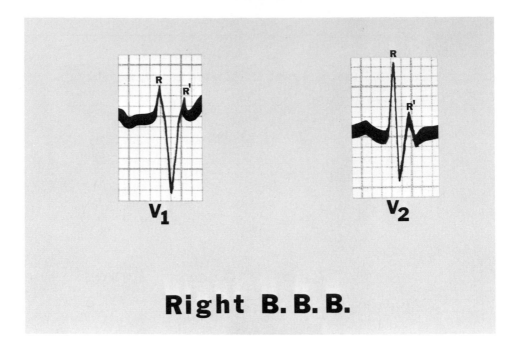

Right B. B. B.

If there is an R,R' in V_1 or V_2, this is Right Bundle Block.

With a wide _____ (and a diagnosis of B.B.B.) one checks the right and left chest leads for R,R'.

QRS

Then if there is an R,R' in V_1 or V_2 this is probably a _____ Bundle Branch Block.

Right

In Right Bundle Branch Block the _____ ventricle is depolarizing slightly later than the left ventricle, so the R' in the above illustration represents the delayed depolarization of the *right* ventricle.

right

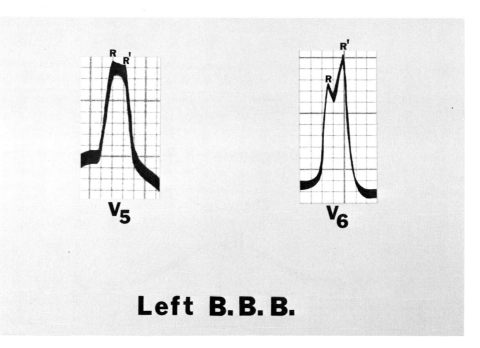

Left B.B.B.

With a Bundle Branch Block an R,R′ in the left chest leads means that Left Bundle Block is present, and the R′ represents delayed depolarization of the *left* ventricle.

The left chest leads are V_5 and V_6 and the sensor electrode is over the left _____ in both leads.   ventricle

Occasionally the R,R′ will be seen only as a notch in the wide _____ in V_5 or V_6.   QRS

In Left Bundle Branch Block the _____ ventricle fires   right
before the left ventricle, so the first portion of the wide
QRS represents right ventricular depolarization.

   NOTE: Compare and make a mental note of the
   characteristic Right and Left Bundle Branch Block
   patterns on these two facing pages, for it is important that
   you are able to distinguish these patterns by sight.

   NOTE: Blocks of either of the two subdivisions of the Left
   Bundle Branch are referred to as *Hemiblocks,* and they are
   explained in detail beginning on page 245.

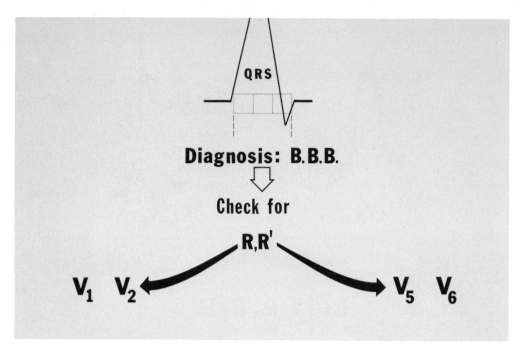

Remember, if there is a wide QRS (3 small squares), identify which Bundle Branch is blocked by checking the left and right chest leads.

To have Bundle Branch Block the QRS must be at least _____ of a second in duration. Just for smiles, let's identify the type of B.B.B. in the illustration on page 149.

.12

NOTE: In some individuals a Bundle Branch Block conduction pattern will not become evident until a certain rapid rate has been reached. When a Bundle Branch Block pattern due to aberrant conduction occurs only at a certain rate this is called "critical rate" Bundle Branch Block. Review NOTE, page 149.

The R,R' pattern may occur in only one chest _____. It is often difficult to see the R' but it can usually be found in V_1, V_2, or in V_5, V_6.

lead

NOTE: Occasionally one can see an R,R' in a QRS of normal duration. This is called "Incomplete" B.B.B.

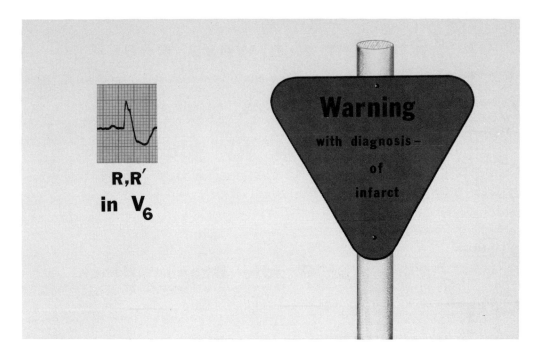

R,R′
in V₆

Warning

with diagnosis –

of

infarct

IMPORTANT: With *Left Bundle Branch Block* one cannot accurately diagnose infarction on EKG.

NOTE: With Left Bundle Branch Block the left ventricle fires late, so the first portion of the QRS complex represents right ventricular activity. Therefore we cannot identify Q waves originating from the left ventricle (which signify infarction), because they will be buried in the widened QRS.

The EKG should be studied for signs of infarction as usual with a _____ Bundle Branch Block.   Right

NOTE: With Left Bundle Branch Block other studies are needed to verify the presence of a suspected acute myocardial infarction.

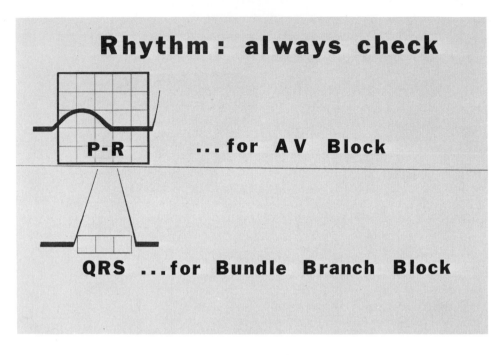

Remember that you must always check* the duration of the P-R intervals and the QRS complex when routinely checking Rhythm.

You must always check* the P-R intervals on all EKG's. Because if any is prolonged more than one large square, then there is some kind of _____ Block present (and, of course, look for dropped QRS's which indicate that a 2° or 3° AV Block is present).

AV

The QRS width must also be checked* on all EKG's, for if it is prolonged there is a _____ _____ Block.

Bundle Branch

> NOTE: Check* the P-R intervals and the QRS width when scrutinizing the rhythm on any EKG. This should be part of your normal routine. The sudden appearance of an AV Block or Bundle Branch Block often indicates impending myocardial infarction.

> NOTE: *Hemiblocks* are explained under Infarction on pages 245–254. A Hemiblock is a block of one of the two divisions ("fascicles") of the Left Bundle Branch.

*"Check" can mean careful *observation* in an emergency situation, or even with random bedside tracings or monitor displays. However, when providing a clinical interpretation, the durations of the P-R intervals and the QRS complex are accurately documented in hundredths of a second.

Bundle Branch Block

Vector : ?

Ventricular Hypertrophy?

The Mean QRS Vector (Axis) and ventricular hypertrophy cannot be accurately calculated in the presence of Bundle Branch Block.

NOTE: Because the Mean QRS Vector represents the general direction of the simultaneous depolarization of the ventricles, it is very difficult to represent such a vector in B.B.B. because the ventricles are firing out of phase, and there are really two separate (right and left) ventricular vectors.

The criteria for ventricular hypertrophy are based on a normal QRS. Bundle Branch Block produces large QRS deflections because each ventricle does not have the (usual) simultaneous electrical opposition by depolarization from the other ventricle. Therefore the EKG diagnosis of _____ hypertrophy should be very   ventricular guarded with B.B.B.

NOTE: In the presence of B.B.B., *atrial* hypertrophy may be diagnosed as per usual.

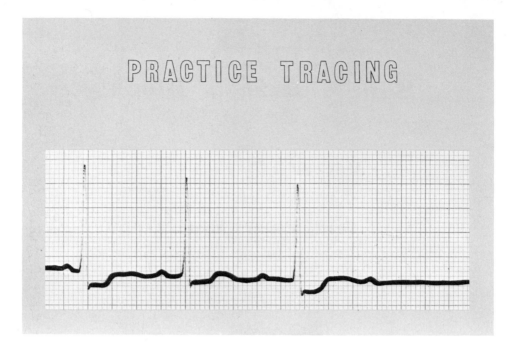

PRACTICE TRACING

An examining physician noted that this patient had an irregular pulse. He was surprised to feel three pulse beats and then a pause. This pattern repeated over and over.

A casual look at all P-R intervals reveals that the last cycle has a P-R interval which is longer than .2 sec., so we suspect some kind of _____ Block.

AV

After the last cycle, we note a lone _____ wave with no QRS response.

P

By close examination we note that the P-R interval is normal at first but becomes progressively longer with each succeeding cycle. We now suspect _____ phenomenon, which is a type of 2° AV Block.

Wenckebach

NOTE: Before you go on, take a little time and slowly review the illustrations on pages 135 to 156.

NOTE: Review Rhythm by turning to the **Personal Quick Reference Sheets** at the end of this book on pages 282 to 285. Also establish your routine methodology (page 280).

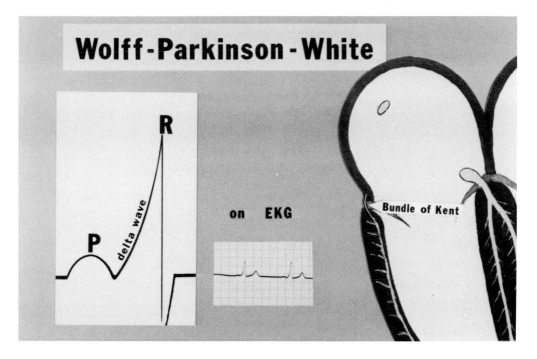

In some individuals an accessory pathway "short circuits" the (usual) delay of ventricular stimulation, causing premature ventricular depolarization represented as a delta wave.

The accessory Bundle of _____ is said to provide ventricular "pre-excitation" in Wolff-Parkinson-White Syndrome.

Kent

The delta wave causes an apparent "shortened" P-R interval and "lengthened" QRS. The delta wave actually represents _____ stimulation to an area of the ventricles.

premature

> NOTE: W.P.W. syndrome is very important because persons with such an accessory conduction path can have paroxysmal tachycardia of two mechanisms:
> re-entry—ventricular depolarization may immediately re-stimulate the atria via this accessory conduction pathway in a retrograde fashion causing a theoretical circus re-entry loop.
> rapid conduction—supraventricular tachycardia (including atrial flutter or atrial fibrillation) may be rapidly conducted to the ventricles 1:1 through this accessory pathway.

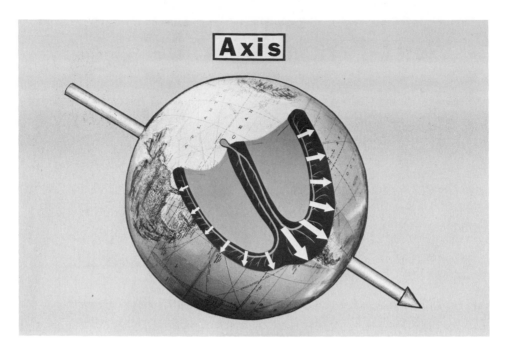

Axis refers to the direction of depolarization which spreads throughout the heart to stimulate the myocardium to contract.

NOTE: The axis around which the earth rotates has nothing to do with electrocardiography, but we can borrow the large arrow ("Axis") in this picture.

Electrical _____ of the muscle cells of the heart proceeds in a certain direction.

stimulation (depolarization)

Axis refers to the _____ of the electrical stimulus of depolarization.

direction

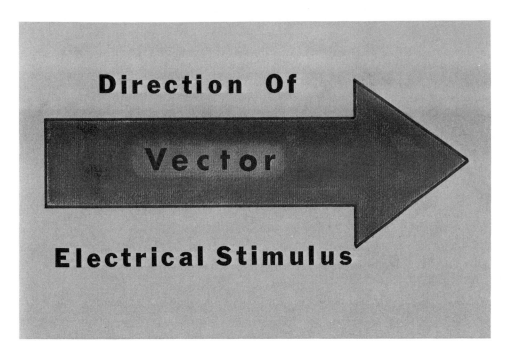

To demonstrate the direction in which depolarization is moving, we use a "vector" which is an arrow.

We can demonstrate the general direction of this electrical path by a _____.   vector

This vector shows the _____ in which most   direction
of the electrical stimulus is traveling.

When interpreting EKG's, a vector shows the direction of
electrical _____.   stimulation
                                                                  (depolarization)

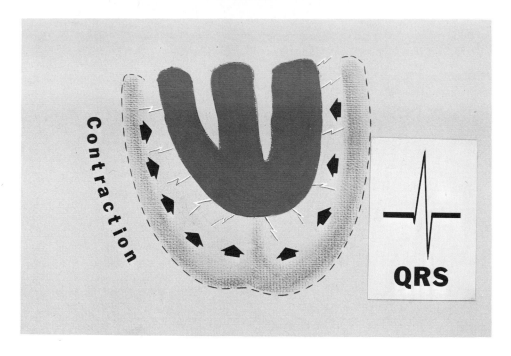

The QRS complex represents the electrical stimulation (and contraction) of the ventricles.

The _____ complex represents the simultaneous stimulation (depolarization) of both ventricles.   QRS

Ventricular depolarization and _____ can be said to be nearly coincident (but we know contraction lasts longer).   contraction

Depolarization of the ventricles and their subsequent contraction is represented by the QRS _____.   complex

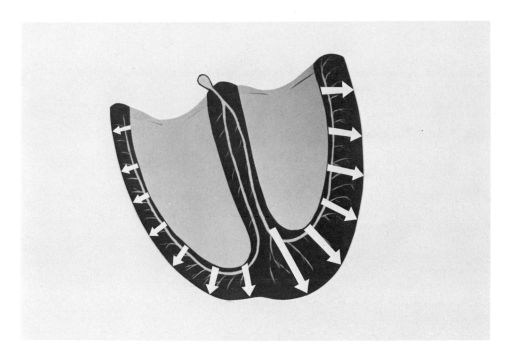

We can use small vectors to demonstrate ventricular depolarization which begins in the endocardium (inner lining) and proceeds through the ventricular wall.

NOTE: Once depolarization is beyond the AV Node, the ventricular conduction system transmits this electrical impulse to the ventricles with great speed. In this way ventricular depolarization begins within the endocardial (lining) surface and proceeds through the thickness of the ventricular wall in all areas at the same time (note small vectors as shown).

The electrical impulse of depolarization is transmitted to all areas of the endocardium (lining of both ventricles) with such great speed that _____ ventricular depolarization generally begins at the level of the endocardium in all areas at the same time.

Depolarization of the ventricles, therefore, essentially proceeds from the _____ to the outside endocardium surface through the full thickness of the ventricular wall in all areas at once.

NOTE: Notice that the left ventricular wall has larger vectors. Also, the septum depolarizes from left to right (not shown).

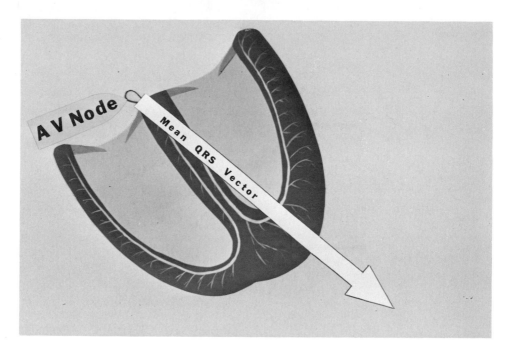

If we add up all the small vectors of ventricular depolarization (considering both direction and magnitude), we have one large "Mean QRS Vector" which represents the general direction of ventricular depolarization.

The origin of the Mean QRS Vector is always the

_____.   AV Node

So no matter where the Mean QRS _____ points, the   Vector
tail is the AV Node.

Because the vectors representing the depolarization of the
left ventricle are larger, the Mean QRS Vector points
slightly toward the left _____.   ventricle

> NOTE: Let me digress to explain that a vector really
> represents direction *and magnitude* (of depolarization), but
> to minimize confusion only direction has been mentioned
> until now. Vectors of larger magnitude will be represented
> by larger arrows; however, some authors use a larger
> number of identical-sized vectors to show greater
> magnitude.

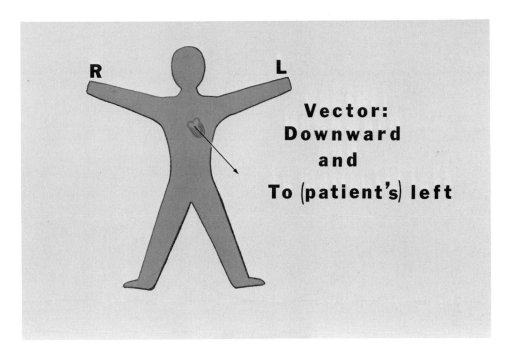

Thus the Mean QRS Vector normally points downward and to the patient's left side.

The ventricles are in the left side of the chest and angle downward and toward the _____.

left

The _____ _____ Vector points downward and toward the patient's left side.

Mean QRS

NOTE: From now on "Vector" (capital "V") will imply the Mean QRS Vector. Visualize the Vector over the patient's chest and remember that it always begins in the AV Node.

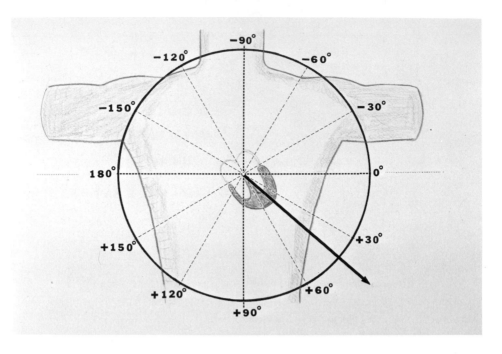

The position of the Mean QRS Vector is noted in degrees within a circle drawn over the patient's chest.

We can locate the position of the Mean QRS Vector within a
large _____ around the heart.   circle

The center of the circle is the _____.   AV Node

The Mean QRS Vector normally points downward and to the
left, or between 0 and _____ degrees.   +90
                                                                  (don't forget
                                                                     the +)

NOTE: The "Axis" of the heart is simply the Mean QRS
Vector when located by degrees in the frontal plane. For
example, the axis of the heart in the above illustration is
about +40 degrees. Review the illustration and note that
0° is on the patient's left, horizontally, and the lower half
of the circle is "positive" degrees, while the top half is
"negative" degrees.

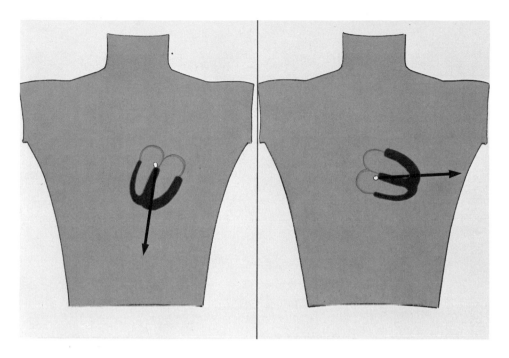

If the heart is displaced, the Vector is also displaced in the same direction. The AV Node is always the tail of the Vector.

If the heart is displaced toward the _____, the Mean QRS Vector points to the right.

right

In very obese people the diaphragm is pushed up (and also the heart), so the Mean QRS Vector may point directly to the _____ (horizontal).

left

The tail of this Vector is always the _____.

AV Node

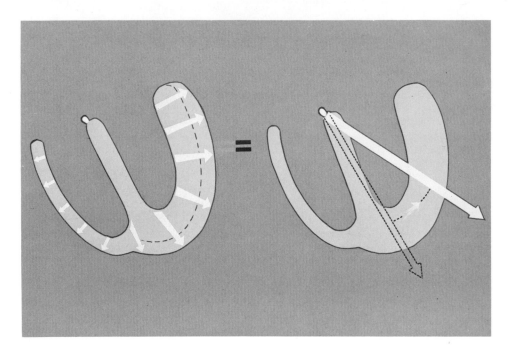

With hypertrophy (enlargement) of one ventricle, the greater electrical activity on the hypertrophied side displaces the vector toward that side.

A hypertrophied ventricle has greater
_____ activity.   electrical

. . . so the Mean QRS Vector deviates toward the
_____ side.   hypertrophied

NOTE: The hypertrophied ventricle has more (and larger) vectors which draw the Mean QRS Vector in that direction.

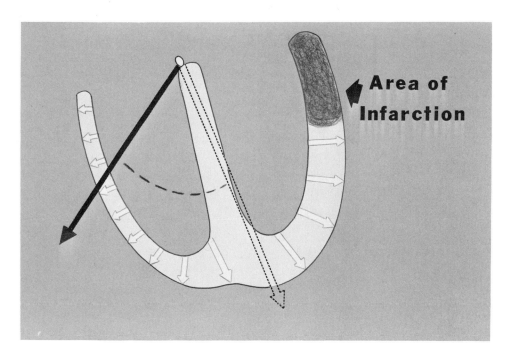

Area of Infarction

In myocardial infarction there is a necrotic (dead) area of the heart that has lost its blood supply and does not conduct an electrical stimulus.

NOTE: Myocardial infarction occurs when a branch of one of the coronary arteries (the only source of blood supply that the heart has) becomes occluded. The area supplied by this blocked coronary artery has no blood supply and becomes electrically dead.

In myocardial infarction (i.e., a coronary occlusion) there is an area in the heart which has no _____ supply. This infarcted area is electrically silent, and therefore has no vectors.

blood

Since there is no electrical activity in the direction of this infarcted area, the Mean QRS Vector tends to point away from it, as there are no _____ in that area (i.e., the vectors in the opposite direction are unopposed).

vectors

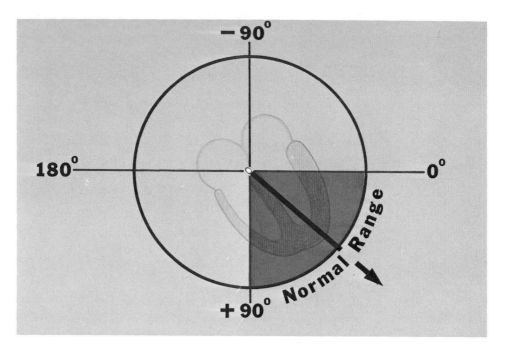

Now you understand why the Mean QRS Vector gives valuable information about cardiac function. "Axis" is the Vector when given in degrees.

The Mean QRS Vector should point downward to the
_____ left or in the 0 to +90 degree range   patient's
(Normal Axis).

The Mean QRS Vector gives us valuable information about
the _____ of the heart,   position

. . . and gives insight into ventricular
_____ and myocardial   hypertrophy
_____.   infarction

NOTE: The Mean QRS Vector tends to point <u>toward</u>
<u>ventricular hypertrophy</u> and <u>away from infarction</u>. As you
can see, these basic principles of Axis are so logical and
easy to understand, that one should employ this useful
diagnostic* tool whenever a twelve lead EKG is available.

*The very backbone of the diagnosis of Hemiblocks is based on changes in Axis.

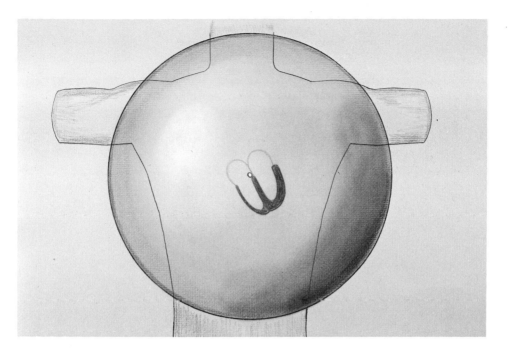

To determine the direction of the Vector, visualize a sphere surrounding the heart with the AV Node at the center of the sphere.

Visualize a large ———————— surrounding the heart.   sphere

The ———————— is the center of the sphere.   AV Node

> NOTE: The Mean QRS Vector will have the AV Node at its tail, and the tip of the arrow will touch somewhere on the surface of this hypothetical sphere.

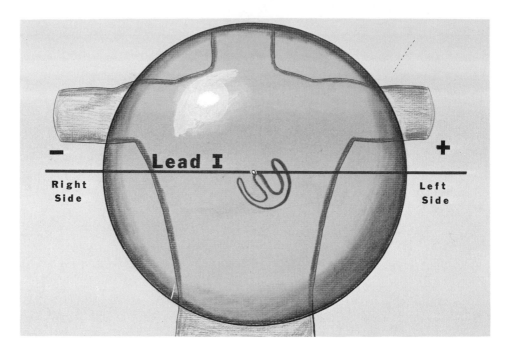

With the sphere in mind, consider lead I (left arm with the positive electrode, right arm with the negative).

Lead I uses the right and left _____ for monitoring.   arms

Introducing lead I into the sphere, the patient's left side
(left arm) is _____.   positive

In lead I the right arm is _____.   negative

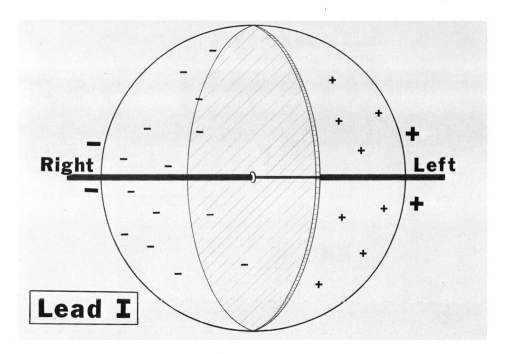

With lead I, the *patient's* left hand side of the sphere is positive and the right half negative.

We can now consider the sphere in two _____.   halves

The patient's right half of the sphere is _____.   negative

Remember that we are considering only lead ____ at this   I
time.

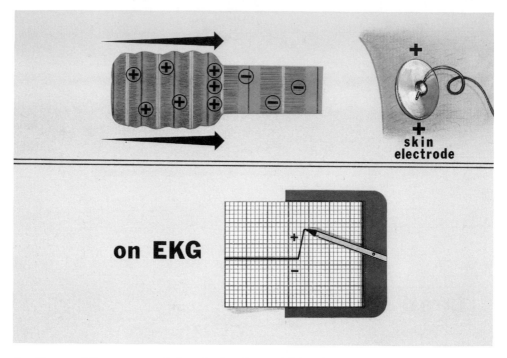

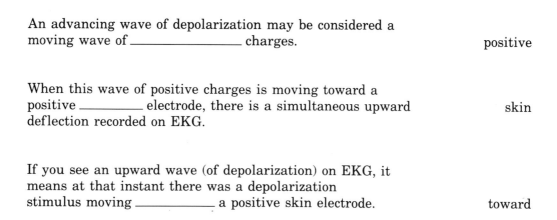

As the positive wave of depolarization within the myocardial cells moves toward a positive (skin) electrode, there is a positive (upward) deflection recorded on EKG.

An advancing wave of depolarization may be considered a moving wave of _____ charges.

positive

When this wave of positive charges is moving toward a positive _____ electrode, there is a simultaneous upward deflection recorded on EKG.

skin

If you see an upward wave (of depolarization) on EKG, it means at that instant there was a depolarization stimulus moving _____ a positive skin electrode.

toward

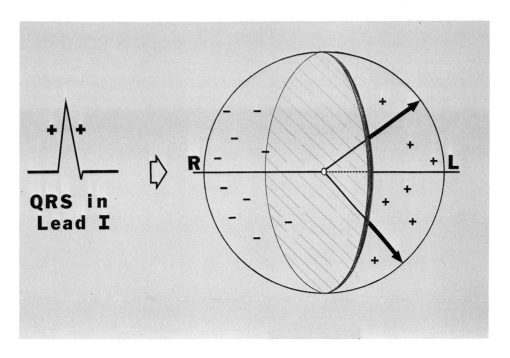

If the QRS complex is POSITIVE (mainly upward) in lead I, the Mean QRS Vector is pointing somewhere into the patient's *left* half of the sphere.

Obtain an EKG tracing and check the _____ complex in lead I.   QRS

> NOTE: We check the QRS complex because it represents ventricular depolarization on the EKG tracing.

If the QRS in lead I is mainly upward, it is _____ (positive or negative),   positive

. . . and if the QRS is positive in lead I, then the Mean QRS Vector points positively or into the _____ half of   left
the sphere (toward that positive skin electrode on the patient's left arm).

> NOTE: This point becomes more clear if you go back and review the preceding page in its entirety.

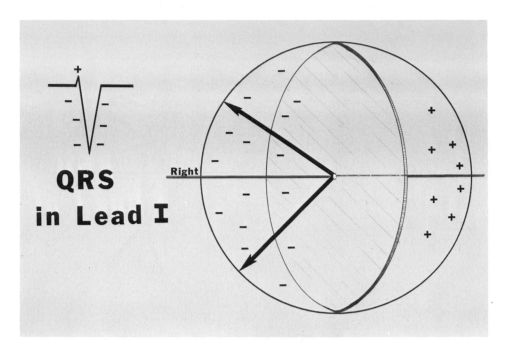

QRS in Lead I

Still considering lead I on the tracing, if the QRS is mainly *negative* (downward), the Vector points to the patient's right side.

In lead I if the QRS complex is mainly below the baseline it is _____ (positive or negative).

negative

Now checking the lead I sphere surrounding the patient, a Vector pointing to the negative half of the sphere points to the patient's _____ side.

right

If the QRS in lead I is mainly negative, then the Mean _____ Vector points to the patient's right side (away from the positive electrode on the patient's left arm).

QRS

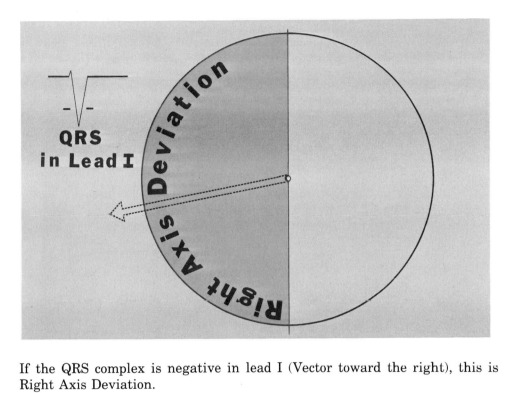

If the QRS complex is negative in lead I (Vector toward the right), this is Right Axis Deviation.

If the Mean QRS Vector points toward the right, we would expect the QRS complex in lead I to be _____.

negative

If the Mean QRS Vector points to the patient's right side (to the right of a vertical line drawn through the AV Node), this is Right _____ Deviation.

Axis

So if the QRS complex is negative in lead ____, this means that there is Right Axis Deviation (R.A.D.).

I

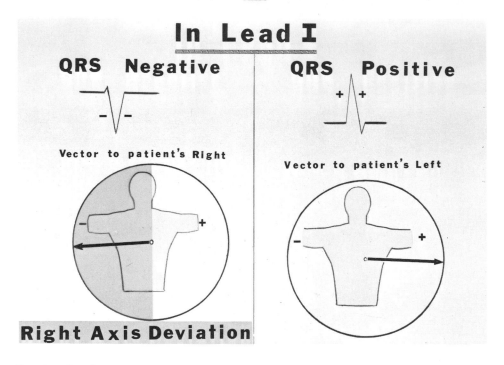

In Lead **I**

QRS Negative | QRS Positive

Vector to patient's Right | Vector to patient's Left

Right Axis Deviation

By simple observation we can tell whether the Mean QRS Vector points to the left or right side of the patient.

Lead _____ is the best lead for detecting Right Axis Deviation.

I

If the QRS complex is positive in lead I (which it usually is), this means there is no R.A.D. because the Vector is pointing to the _____ side of the patient.

left

In lead I the patient's left arm carries the _____ electrode.

positive

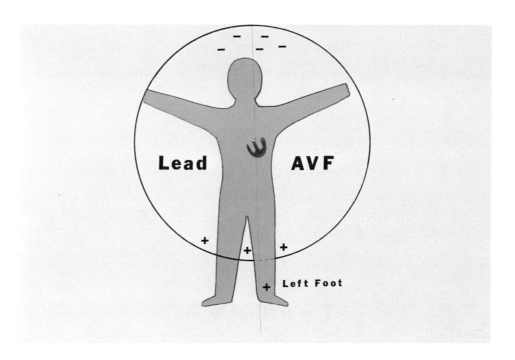

Lead AVF has a positive electrode on the left foot. Imagine a sphere around the patient for lead AVF.

Forget about the lead previously mentioned. We will consider only lead _____ at this time.

AVF

NOTE: We are now going to consider a completely different sphere—that one surrounding the body when we monitor lead AVF on the EKG machine. We will have to re-orient ourselves as to the positive and negative halves of the sphere in AVF.

When we change the EKG machine to monitor lead AVF, the machine makes the sensor of the _____ foot positive.

left

The lower half of this sphere is _____ (positive or negative).

positive

The center of the new sphere is the _____.

AV Node

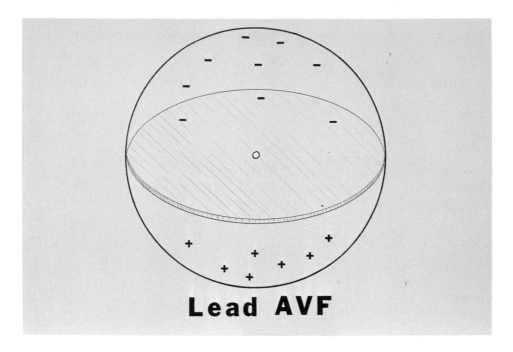

Lead AVF

For AVF the lower half of the sphere is positive, and the upper half is negative.

The upper portion of the sphere (above the AV Node) is
_____ (positive or negative).   negative

The sphere in AVF has two halves, the upper half being
_____, the lower half being   negative
_____.   positive

Below the AV Node the (lead AVF) sphere is
_____. Reoriented now?   positive

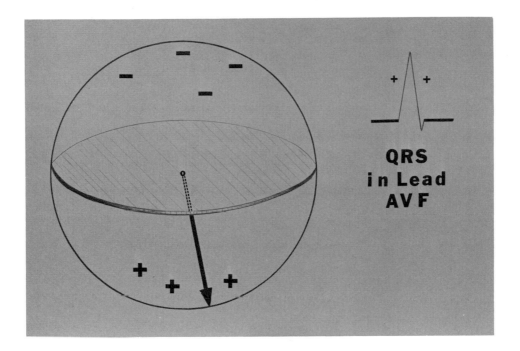

QRS
in Lead
AVF

In lead AVF if the QRS is mainly positive on the tracing, then the Mean QRS Vector points downward.

In lead AVF if the Mean QRS Vector points downward, then the QRS complex on the tracing is _____.

upright or positive

NOTE: Don't get confused just because the positive QRS is upright, and the Vector points downward. You must remember that the Vector is pointing into the positive half of the sphere when the QRS is positive. The lower half of the sphere just happens to be the positive half in lead AVF.

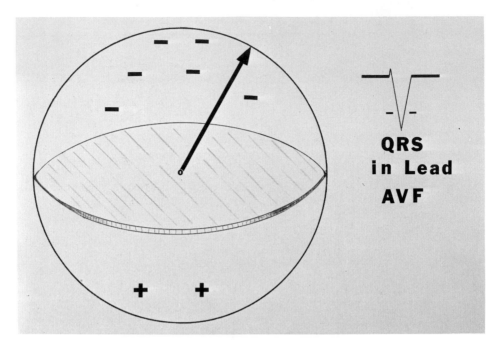

QRS in Lead AVF

In AVF if the QRS is negative, the Vector points upward into the negative half of the sphere.

The _____ of the sphere is the AV Node.

center

The upper half of the (lead AVF) sphere is _____ (positive or negative).

negative

A negative QRS complex in lead AVF tells us that the Mean QRS Vector points _____ into the negative half of the sphere (i.e. it is pointing away from the positive electrode on the left foot).

upward

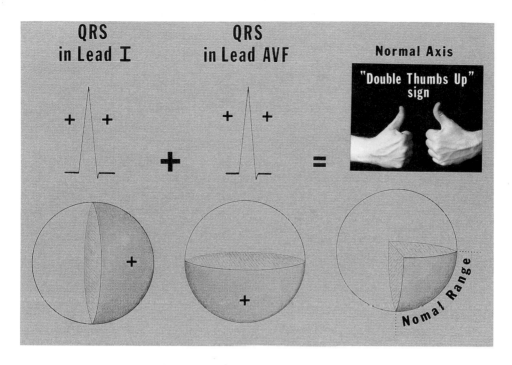

If the QRS is positive in lead I and also positive in AVF, the Vector points downward and to the patient's left (normal range).

A mainly positive QRS in lead I indicates that the Mean QRS Vector points to the _____ side of the patient.

left

A mainly positive QRS complex in lead AVF means that the Vector points _____.

downward

So if the QRS is positive in both leads I and AVF, the Mean QRS _____ must point downward and to the left side of the patient (and it usually does).

Vector

NOTE: The Mean QRS Vector is in the normal range when it points downward to the left, since the ventricles point downward to the patient's left. Remember that when speaking of Vector position, left or right refers to the patient's left or right side. If the QRS is upright in I and AVF, (the "double thumbs up sign"), then the Vector ("Axis") is within the normal range.

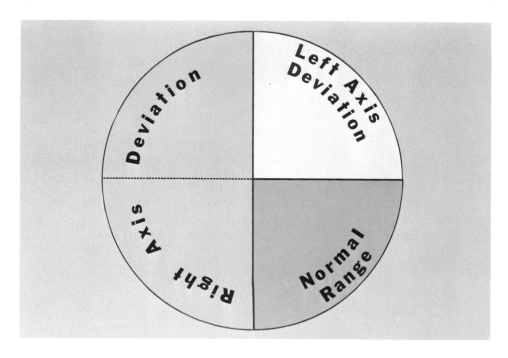

These are the four possible axis quadrants where the Mean QRS Vector may point. Visualize this large circle on the patient's chest.

If the Vector points upward (from the AV Node) and to the patient's left, this is Left _____ Deviation (L.A.D.).

Axis

If the Vector points to the patient's right side, this is _____ Axis Deviation (R.A.D.).

Right

If the Vector points downward to the patient's left, it is in the _____ range (i.e. Normal Axis).

normal

> NOTE: Remember, Axis is merely the position (i.e. the direction) of the Mean QRS Vector.

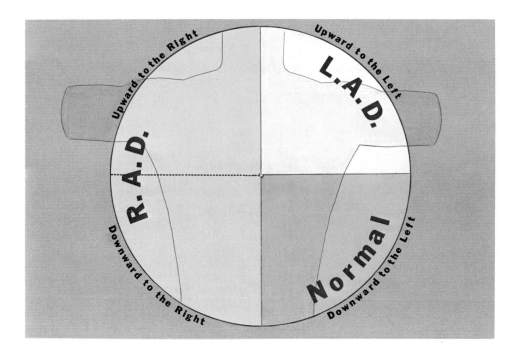

By finding into which axis quadrant the Vector points, we know in which direction ventricular depolarization is going.

NOTE: This is the manner in which you should visualize the four axis quadrants in a large circle (AV Node is center) drawn on the patient's chest. On some EKG charts you may see such a circle into which this Mean QRS Vector is drawn (in the frontal plane).

The upper left quadrant represents _____ Axis Deviation (L.A.D.).

Left

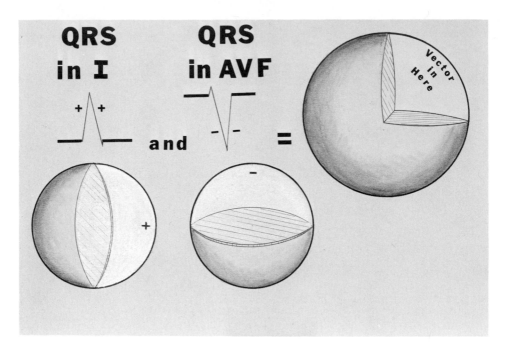

If the QRS is *positive* in lead I, and *negative* in AVF, that places the Vector in the upper left quadrant.

If the QRS in lead I is upright, the Vector points to the patient's _____.

left

If the Vector is pointing upwards, then the QRS in lead AVF is mainly _____ the baseline.

below

If the Vector points upward and to the patient's left, this is Left _____ Deviation (L.A.D.).

Axis

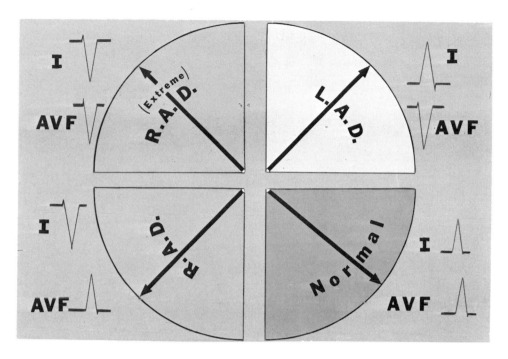

Now by looking at the QRS complex in I and AVF you can locate the Mean QRS Vector in an axis quadrant (in the frontal plane).

Any time the QRS complex is negative in lead I, there is
_____ Axis Deviation (R.A.D.), and when the Vector
points upward and to the patient's right, this is often called
"extreme" Right Axis Deviation.

Right

But if the QRS is positive in lead I and negative in lead
AVF, there is Left Axis _____.

Deviation

If the Mean QRS Vector points downward and to the
patient's left, we would expect the QRS complexes in lead I
and AVF to be mainly _____ (positive or
negative).

positive

NOTE: One can calculate the vector for a portion of a QRS complex (e.g., the initial or terminal .04 sec.) in exactly the same manner as for the Mean QRS Vector.

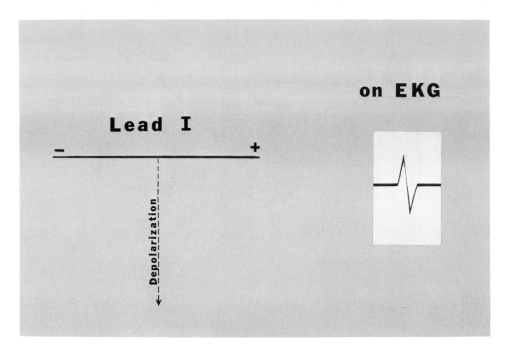

When depolarization proceeds in a direction perpendicular to the orientation of a given lead, the deflection is minimal and/or "isoelectric."

Depolarization, when perpendicular to the orientation of a lead, is directed negligibly toward either sensor, so the recorded deflection is as much negative as positive and is called _____.   isoelectric

The word isoelectric literally means "same voltage," so positive and negative portions of the QRS complex are about _____.   equal

Although the positive and negative deflections of an isoelectric QRS are equal in magnitude, they are generally _____ in the limb leads.   small

NOTE: First, locate the Mean QRS Vector in a given axis quadrant (i.e., Normal, L.A.D., R.A.D., or Extreme R.A.D.). Then, find the lead in which the QRS is most isoelectric, so you can more precisely locate the Vector (Axis). The Axis will be about 90° from the orientation of the most "isoelectric" lead. It is really very easy . . . see next page.

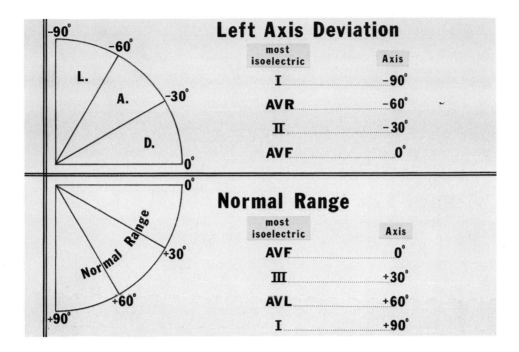

Left Axis Deviation

most isoelectric	Axis
I	−90°
AVR	−60°
II	−30°
AVF	0°

Normal Range

most isoelectric	Axis
AVF	0°
III	+30°
AVL	+60°
I	+90°

It is customary to locate the position of the Vector (Axis) in a more exact way (i.e., in degrees) in the frontal plane: first locate the axis quadrant, and then note the limb lead in which the QRS is most isoelectric.

NOTE: In review: First, locate the appropriate axis quadrant, then to determine the exact position of the Vector (Axis), note the lead where the QRS is most isoelectric.

A patient with Left Axis Deviation would have a Mean QRS Vector of between 0 and _____ degrees (QRS positive in I and negative in AVF).

−90°
(don't forget the negative)

A patient with a Mean QRS Vector in the normal range would have an electrical axis of +30° if the QRS in lead _____ was isoelectric.

III

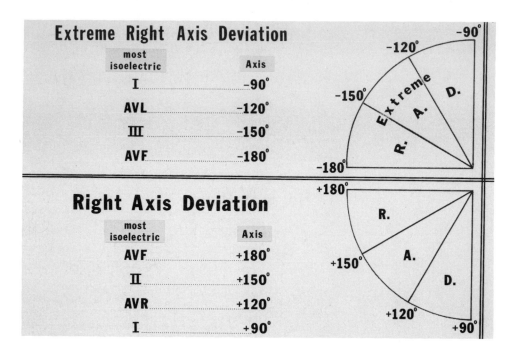

Extreme Right Axis Deviation	
most isoelectric	Axis
I	−90°
AVL	−120°
III	−150°
AVF	−180°

Right Axis Deviation	
most isoelectric	Axis
AVF	+180°
II	+150°
AVR	+120°
I	+90°

The exact position of the Vector (Axis) can be located in a similar way for Right Axis Deviation and Extreme Right Axis Deviation.

NOTE: In each case the axis quadrant is determined, then the lead with the most isoelectric QRS is noted.*

A patient with R.A.D. and an Axis of +150 degrees would probably have a tracing with an isoelectric QRS in lead ____.

II

Finding an Axis of approximately −150° would mean that the Vector is in the quadrant of _____ R.A.D.

Extreme

NOTE: An Axis of 180° is either + or − depending on whether the Vector is in the R.A.D. or Extreme R.A.D. quadrant respectively.

*This is summarized for you (page 286) as your **Personal Quick Reference Sheet**, which is self explanatory.

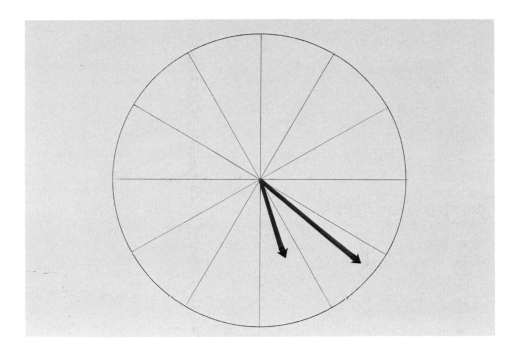

The Axis is often recorded like the hands of a clock, the longer arrow is the Mean QRS Vector, the shorter is the T wave vector.

The T wave has a vector which can be located by employing the same method that we use for locating the _____   QRS Vector.

> NOTE: When the T wave vector and the QRS Vector are separated by 60° or more, this generally signifies pathology.

The T wave vector is usually represented as a _____ arrow than the QRS Vector.   smaller

> NOTE: Axis is often noted in the literature by an "A" as in A +60°, and it may be called "electrical axis."

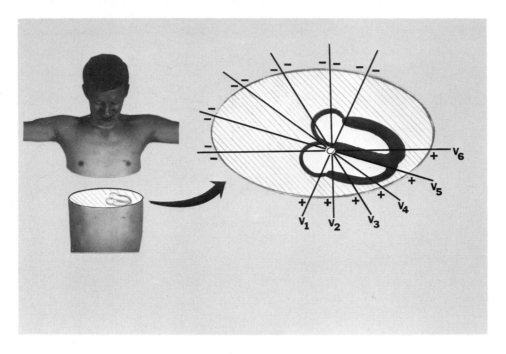

There are three dimensions to the sphere so it is important to note the general position of the Mean QRS Vector in the horizontal plane as well.

The horizontal _____ divides the body into top and   plane
bottom halves.

The chest leads form the _____ plane.   horizontal

NOTE: To determine changes ("rotation") of the Mean
QRS Vector in the horizontal plane, one should examine
the chest leads.

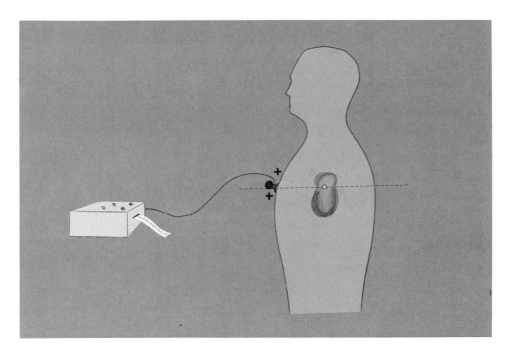

Lead V_2 is obtained by placing an electrode sensor on the chest along the left side of the sternum (at the fourth interspace).

The electrode sensor for lead V_2 is _____   positive
(positive or negative).

> NOTE: The sensor electrode for the chest leads is on a suction cup which is moved to a different position on the chest for each of the six chest leads (which form the horizontal plane). In each case the suction cup sensor is positive.

The position of the sensor for lead V_2 places it in front of
the heart at the fourth interspace to the left
of the _____.   sternum

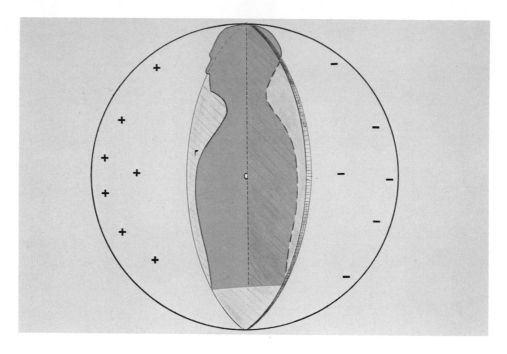

Considering a sphere for lead V_2 we can see that the front half is positive and the back half is negative.

Considering a sphere for lead V_2, we will view the patient from the side, but the _____ of the sphere is still the AV Node.

center

The patient's back is considered _____ (positive or negative) when considering lead V_2.

negative

The front half of the sphere is considered _____ in lead V_2.

positive

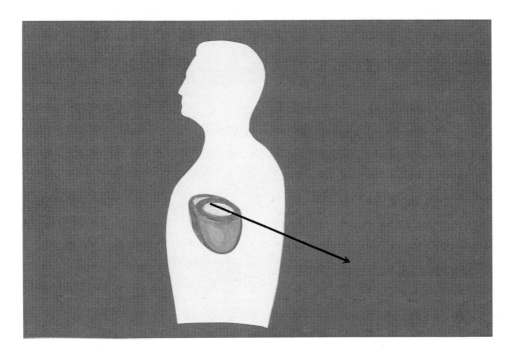

Normally the QRS in lead V_2 is negative, so the Mean QRS Vector points backward because of the (generally) posteriorly positioned thick left ventricle.

On the standard EKG the QRS complex in lead V_2 is usually _____ (or below the baseline).

negative

Therefore the Mean QRS Vector usually points _____ into the negative half of the sphere.

backward

Normally most of the ventricular depolarization is directed away from the positive V_2 electrode, toward the thicker and more posteriorly positioned _____ ventricle.

left

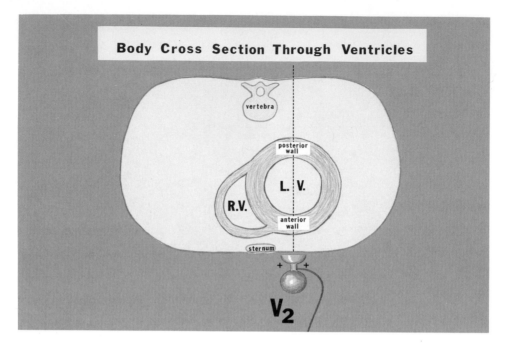

Body Cross Section Through Ventricles

The orientation of V_2 makes it the most important lead for the determination of both Anterior and Posterior Infarctions.

The orientation of lead V_2 projects directly through the anterior wall and the posterior wall of the left
_____.   ventricle

So lead V_2 reflects the most reliable information concerning Anterior Infarction and Posterior Infarction of the _____   left
ventricle.

> NOTE: As you will soon see, both ventricular depolarization and repolarization should be scrutinized in the right chest leads, because subtle vector changes are reflected there by both anterior and posterior infarctions (of the left ventricle).

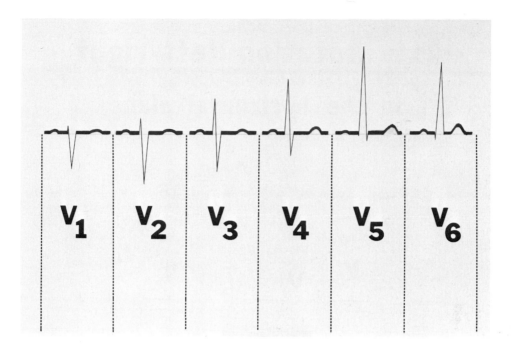

There is a gradual transition from the generally negative QRS in V_1 to the generally positive (upright) QRS in V_6.

The QRS is usually mainly negative in lead V_1, and it is mostly _____ in lead V_6.

positive

If one scans lead V_1 through lead V_6, it is noted that the QRS becomes as much positive as _____ (i.e., isoelectric) in lead V_3 or V_4. This is known as the *transitional zone.*

negative

> NOTE: You will recall that an isoelectric QRS is 90° away from Mean QRS Vector. So a shift ("rotation") of the Vector in the horizontal plane (of the chest leads) is reflected as a change in position of the "transitional" (isoelectric) QRS in the chest leads.

Axis Rotation (left/right)
in the horizontal plane

"Counter-clockwise" rotation V₁ V₂ Normal Range V₃ V₄ "Clockwise" rotation V₅ V₆

Rotation of the Vector in the horizontal plane is noted in terms of *clockwise* (toward the patient's left) or *counter-clockwise* (toward the patient's right) rotation.

NOTE: With the AV Node as the anchored tail of the Mean QRS Vector, we can determine rotation of the Vector in the hoizontal plane. When the isoelectric "transitional" QRS has moved to the patient's left, into leads V_5 or V_6, this is called *clockwise rotation*. If we see a transitional QRS (i.e. isoelectric QRS) in right chest leads V_1 or V_2, this is *counter-clockwise rotation*.* Anatomically, the heart is not capable of much movement in the horizontal plane, but we do know that the Vector tends to shift toward Ventricular Hypertrophy and away from Infarction, so this is exceptionally valuable information.

NOTE: Axis *deviation* is in the frontal plane, while *rotation* is in the horizontal plane. Review Axis by turning to the **P**ersonal **Q**uick **R**eference **S**heets at the end of this book on page 286, and note the simplified methodology on page 280.

---

*I would have preferred naming these Vector shifts "leftward" and "rightward" since they don't relate well to my clocks, but since Medicine reveres tradition we will respect the conventional terminology.

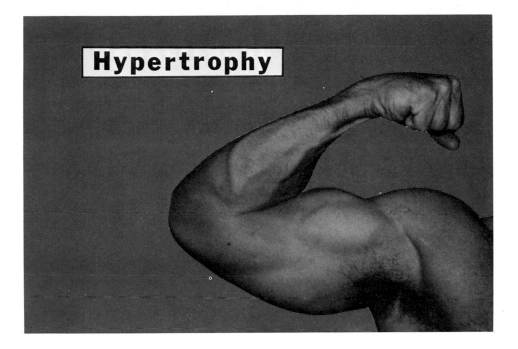

Hypertrophy usually refers to an increase in size, and when relating to muscle this term refers to increase in muscle mass.

Note: This picture is the arm of a weight lifting enthusiast. I had contemplated using a picture of my own arm, but I soon abandoned the idea because I would then have to title this section "hypotrophy" (if there is such a word).

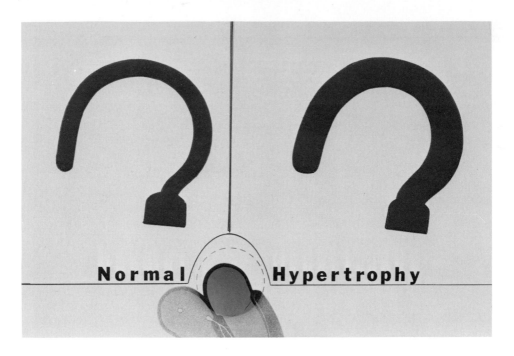

Normal / Hypertrophy

Hypertrophy of a chamber of the heart refers to an increase in the thickness of the wall of that chamber, but some dilation is always present.

Hypertrophy of a chamber of the heart means that the muscular wall of that chamber has dilated and thickened beyond _____ thickness.

normal

Hypertrophy may increase the volume which the _____ contains, and the wall of that chamber is usually thicker than normal.

chamber

The increase in the muscular thickness of the wall of a given chamber of the heart may be diagnosed on _____.

EKG

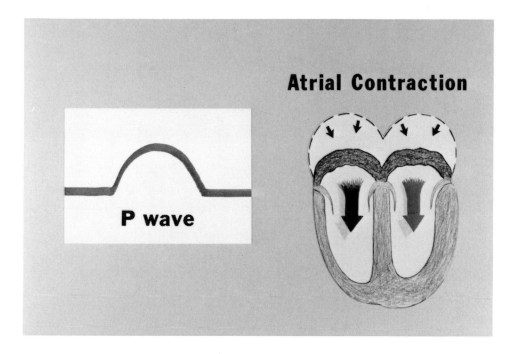

Since the P wave represents the contraction of both atria, we examine the P wave for evidence of atrial hypertrophy.

The depolarization of both atria causes their _____.   contraction

The depolarization of both atria is recorded on EKG as a _____ wave.   P

Signs of _____ hypertrophy can be noted by   atrial
examining the P wave on the EKG tracing.

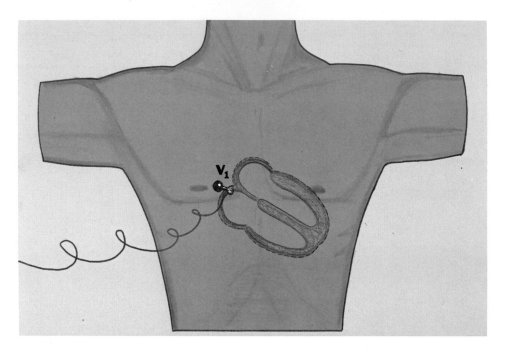

Lead V_1 is directly over the atria, so the P wave in V_1 is our best source of information about atrial enlargement.

The sensor electrode which is placed on the chest when recording lead V_1 is considered _____ (positive or negative).

positive

Lead V_1 is recorded by placing an electrode just to the right of the sternum and in the 4th interspace; this places our suction cup sensor directly over the _____.

atria

Because this electrode is closest to the atria, lead V_1 should be the most valuable lead to check for atrial _____.

hypertrophy

So one would expect the P wave in lead _____ to give us the most accurate information about atrial hypertrophy—and it does!

V_1

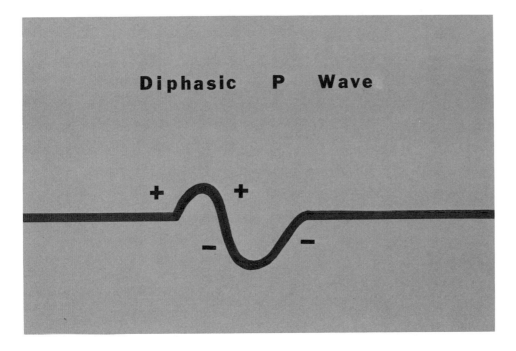

With atrial hypertrophy, the P wave is diphasic (both positive *and* negative).

A wave which has both positive and negative portions is
called a _____ wave (two phase wave).   diphasic

By diphasic we mean that the same wave has deflections
_____ and below the baseline.   above

The diphasic P wave is characteristic of atrial hypertrophy,
but we want to know which _____ is hypertrophied.   atrium

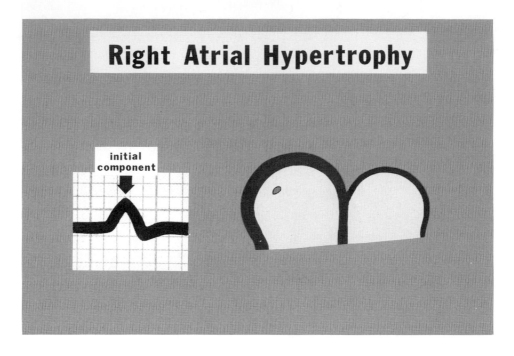

If the initial component of a diphasic P wave (in V_1) is largest, this is *Right Atrial Hypertrophy.*

If the P wave in lead V_1 is _____, then we know
that one of the atria is hypertrophied.

diphasic

If the _____ portion of the diphasic P wave is
the largest of the two phases, then there is Right Atrial
Hypertrophy.

initial

A diphasic P wave in V_1 with a large, often peaked, initial
component tells us that this patient's _____ atrium is
thicker and probably more dilated than his left.

right

NOTE: If the height of the P wave in any of the limb
leads exceeds $2^1/_2$ mm (even if it's *not* diphasic), suspect
Right Atrial Hypertrophy.

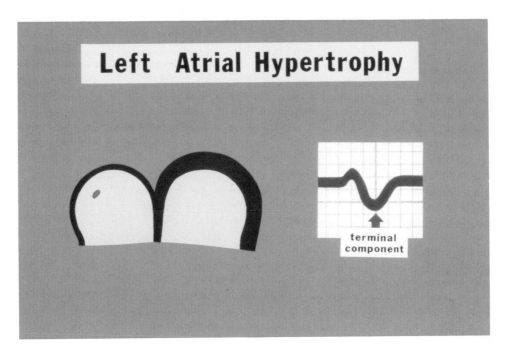

If the terminal portion of a diphasic P wave in V_1 is large and wide, there is
Left Atrial Hypertrophy.

A patient who has hypertrophy of the left atrium because
the mitral (outflow) valve is stenosed* will have a diphasic
P wave in lead ____. V_1

The _____ component of this patient's P wave in   terminal
V_1 is the largest component.

The terminal component of a diphasic P wave in lead V_1 is
usually _____ (positive or negative).   negative

*This narrowing of the lumen of the mitral valve is but one of many potential causes of left atrial
  hypertrophy.

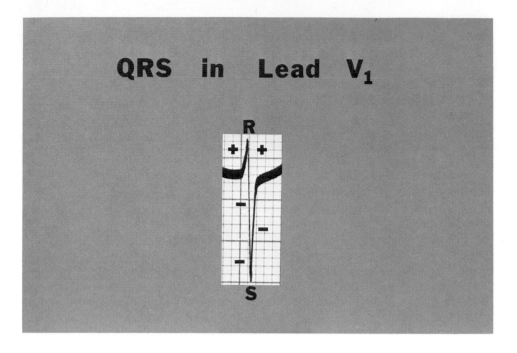

Considering the QRS complex in V_1, the S wave is normally larger than the R wave.

The QRS complex represents ventricular activation, so we would expect it to reflect some indications of the presence of _____ hypertrophy.

ventricular

In lead V_1 the QRS complex is mainly negative, and the _____ wave is therefore usually very short.

R

NOTE: The V_1 electrode is positive. Ventricular depolarization moves downward to the patient's left side and posteriorly (the thicker left ventricle is more posteriorly located). Because ventricular depolarization is moving *AWAY* from the V_1 (positive) electrode, the QRS in V_1 is usually mainly negative. Remember that the Positive depolarization wave moving toward a Positive electrode records a Positive deflection on the EKG tracing. Similarly, depolarization moving *away* from a positive electrode records negatively.

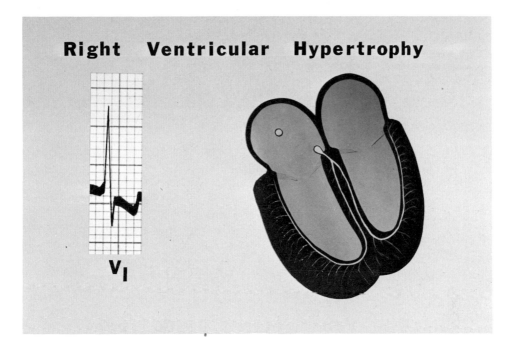

Right Ventricular Hypertrophy

V_1

However, in *Right Ventricular Hypertrophy* there is a large R wave in V_1.

In Right Ventricular Hypertrophy there is a large _____ wave in lead V_1.

R

NOTE: With Right Ventricular Hypertrophy the wall of the right ventricle is very thick, so there is much more (positive) depolarization (and more vectors) toward the (positive) V_1 electrode. We would therefore expect the QRS in lead V_1 to be more positive (upward) than usual.

The S wave in lead V_1 is _____ than the R wave in Right Ventricular Hypertrophy.

smaller

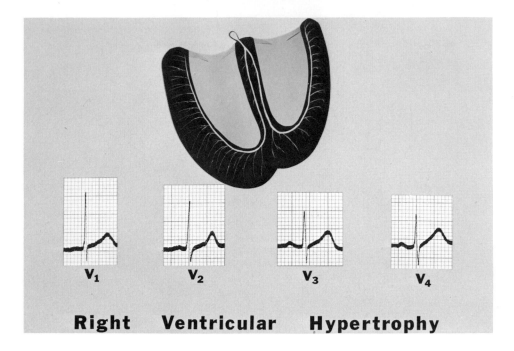

Right   Ventricular   Hypertrophy

In Right Ventricular Hypertrophy, the large R wave of V_1 gets progressively smaller in V_2, V_3, V_4, etc.

When Right Ventricular Hypertrophy is present, there is a large R wave in lead _____ which becomes progressively smaller in chest leads V_2, V_3, and V_4.

V_1

The progressive decrease in the height of the _____ wave is gradual, proceeding from the right chest leads to the left chest leads.

R

NOTE: The enlarged right ventricle adds more vectors toward the right side, so there is Right Axis Deviation (in the frontal plane) and often rightward ("counter-clockwise") rotation of the Vector in the horizontal plane. Visualize the reason for these Vector shifts, and you will comprehend the criteria more clearly.

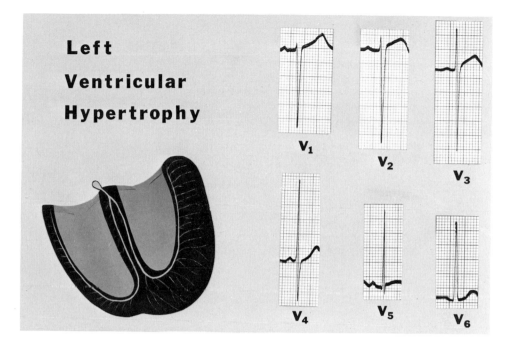

Left Ventricular Hypertrophy

V₁   V₂   V₃   V₄   V₅   V₆

In *Left Ventricular Hypertrophy,* the left ventricular wall is very thick causing great QRS deflections (chest leads).

The wall of the _____ ventricle is normally the thickest of all heart chambers.

left

Hypertrophy of the left ventricle causes QRS complexes which are exaggerated in both height and depth, especially in the _____ leads.

chest

NOTE: Normally the S wave in lead V₁ is deep. But with Left Ventricular Hypertrophy even more depolarization is going downward to the patient's left—away from the positive V₁ electrode. Therefore the S wave will be even deeper in V₁. There will be Left Axis Deviation, and often the Vector will be displaced to the left ("clockwise" rotation) in the horizontal plane. Visualize and understand the reason for these shifts of the Vector. Lasting knowledge results from understanding.

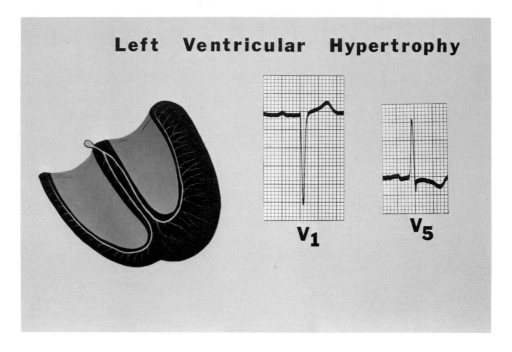

Left Ventricular Hypertrophy

V_1 V_5

With Left Ventricular Hypertrophy there is a large S in V_1 and a large R in V_5.

With Left Ventricular Hypertrophy there is a very tall _____ wave in lead V_5.

R

NOTE: Lead V_5 is over the Left Ventricle, so the increased depolarization is going toward the electrode of V_5 when there is L.V.H. This results in more (positive) depolarization going toward the (positive) electrode of V_5, producing a very tall R wave in that lead.

In Left Ventricular Hypertrophy there is a very tall R wave in _____, and this excessive depolarization moving away from the V_1 electrode produces a deep S wave in lead V_1.

V_5

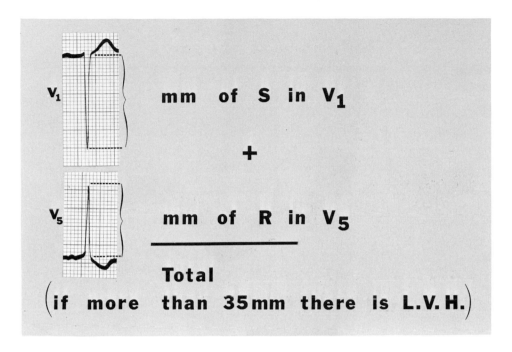

$$\frac{mm \ of \ S \ in \ V_1 \ + \ mm \ of \ R \ in \ V_5}{Total}$$

(if more than 35mm there is L.V.H.)

Depth (in mm) of S in V_1 plus the height of R in V_5 . . . if greater than 35 mm, there is Left Ventricular Hypertrophy.

To check an EKG for Left Ventricular Hypertrophy, one must add the depth of the S wave in V_1 to the height of the _____ wave in V_5.

R

If the depth (in mm) of the S wave in V_1 added to the height of the R wave (in mm) in V_5 is greater than 35, then Left Ventricular _____ is present.

Hypertrophy

NOTE: This addition of the S in V_1 plus the R in V_5 should be routinely checked (mere observation will usually tell) with every twelve lead EKG. When providing a written EKG interpretation, however, one should measure and document the amplitude of these waves in millimeters.

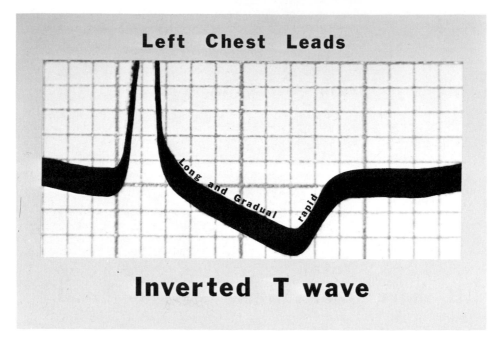

The T wave often shows "Left Ventricular Hypertrophy" characteristics. There is T wave *inversion* and *asymmetry*.

There is a characteristic _____ wave which can usually be seen when Left Ventricular Hypertrophy is present.

T

Since the left chest leads (V_5 or V_6) are over the _____ ventricle, these are ideal leads to check for this T wave which indicates L.V.H.

left

This *inverted* T wave has a gradual downslope and a very steep return to the _____, making it asymmetrical.

baseline

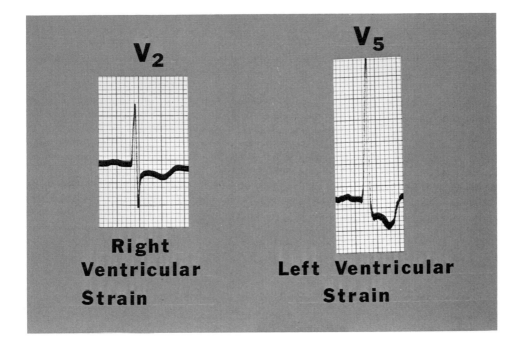

Ventricular hypertrophy may be associated with a strain pattern. With ventricular strain the ST segment becomes depressed and humped.

Ventricular strain is characterized by moderate depression of the _____ segment.

ST

> NOTE: Strain is usually associated with ventricular hypertrophy, which is logical, since a ventricle which is straining against some kind of resistance (e.g., valvular or increased vascular resistance) will become hypertrophied in its attempt to compensate.

Ventricular _____ causes a depressed ST segment which generally curves upward or humps gradually in the middle of the segment.

strain

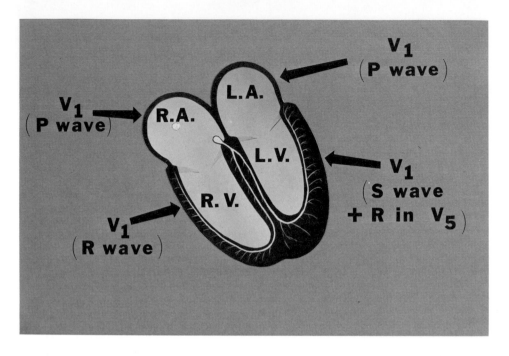

Note that most of the information concerning hypertrophy of heart chambers is gained from V_1.

When routinely reading a 12 lead EKG tracing, you should
check to see if there is _____ of any of   hypertrophy
the chambers.

First, check the P wave in lead V_1 to see if it is
_____.   diphasic

Second, check the R wave in V_1, and then check the S wave
in V_1 and the _____ wave in V_5.   R

> NOTE: Review Hypertrophy by turning to the **P**ersonal
> **Q**uick **R**eference **S**heets at the end of this book on page
> 287 and relate this to the simplified methodology (page
> 280).

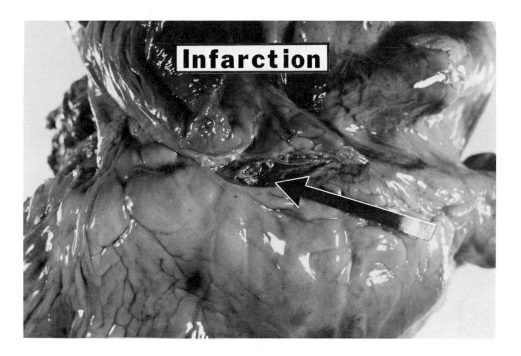

Arteriosclerosis may occlude a coronary artery, or an arteriosclerotic plaque may be the seat of a thrombus which occludes a coronary. Coronary occlusion causes *Myocardial Infarction*.

NOTE: Myocardial Infarction results from an occlusion of a coronary artery. An area of the heart is then without blood supply. This type of occlusion may be relative in that a person with severely narrowed coronary arteries may function well at rest. But with excitement or exertion the rapidly pumping heart demands an increased blood (and oxygen) supply which his coronaries cannot deliver. This type of Myocardial Infarction can be just as serious or deadly as can a classical coronary occlusion.

NOTE: This section is called *Infarction* which infers a complete occlusion of a coronary artery. We can also determine whether a coronary artery is somewhat narrowed, rendering a decreased blood supply to the heart. Therefore keep in mind that we read the electrocardiogram to determine the status of coronary perfusion of the heart. Coronary spasm also plays a role in coronary disease.

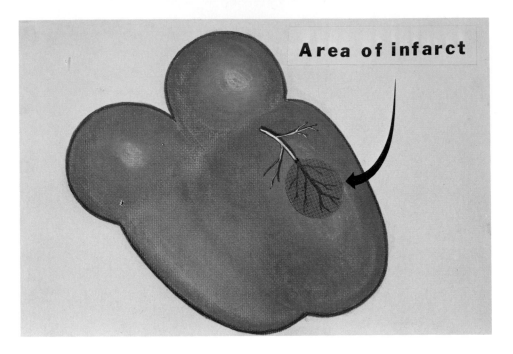

Area of infarct

Myocardial Infarction occurs when a coronary artery supplying the left ventricle becomes occluded, producing an area of myocardium without blood supply.

The terms myocardial infarction, _____ occlusion, and heart attack refer to the same serious phenomenon.

coronary

The heart derives its only blood supply from the _____ arteries, and when a branch of a coronary artery narrows markedly or is blocked, the area of myocardium which this branch supplies is without adequate circulation.

coronary

This "infarcted" area is usually in the left ventricle and serious arrhythmias or _____ may result.

death

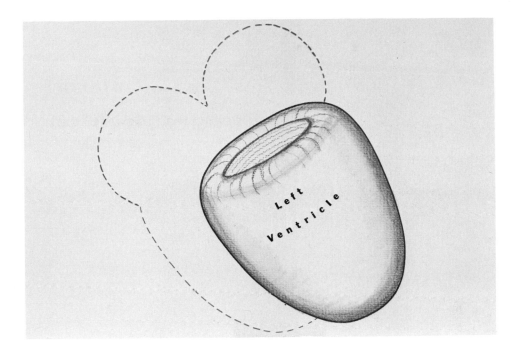

Usually only the thick *left* ventricle suffers myocardial infarction.

The left ventricle is the thickest chamber of the heart; so if the coronary arteries are narrowed, the left ventricle, which needs the greatest blood supply, is the first to suffer from diminished _____ circulation.

coronary

The blood is pumped to all parts of the body by the heavy _____ ventricle.

left

NOTE: When we describe infarcts by location, we are speaking of an area within the left ventricle. Arteries to the left ventricle may send branches to other areas of the heart, so an infarction of the left ventricle can include a small area of another chamber.

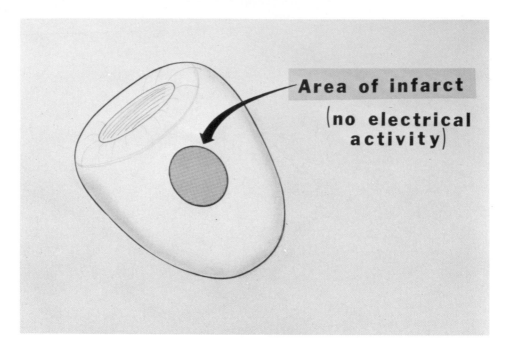

Area of infarct

(no electrical activity)

This infarcted area of the left ventricle with no blood supply is electrically dead and cannot conduct electrical impulses.

Infarctions generally occur within the wall of the left _____.

An area of infarction conducts no _____ impulses because the cells are dead and cannot depolarize normally.

ventricle

electrical

NOTE: This infarcted area produces an electrical void, and the rest of the heart (with an adequate blood supply) functions as usual.

Ischemia

Injury

Infarction

The classical triad of an acute myocardial infarction is "ISCHEMIA," "INJURY," and "INFARCTION," but any of these three may occur alone.

The "three I" triad is the basis for recognizing and diagnosing the signs of _____ infarction.   myocardial

_____ means literally reduced blood, referring to   Ischemia
poor blood supply.

> NOTE: Ischemia, Injury, and Infarction need not all be
> present at once to establish the diagnosis of myocardial
> infarction, but rather provide a good set of criteria to check
> routinely.

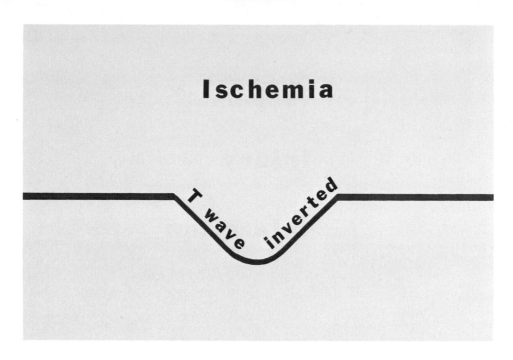

Ischemia (decreased blood supply) is characterized by inverted (upside-down) T waves.

Ischemia means reduced _____ supply (from the coronary arteries) or less than is normally present.

blood

T wave _____ is the characteristic sign of Ischemia and may vary from a slightly flattened or depressed wave to deep inversion.

inversion

Inverted _____ waves may indicate ischemia in the absence of myocardial infarction. There can be a reduced blood supply to the heart without creating an infarction.

T

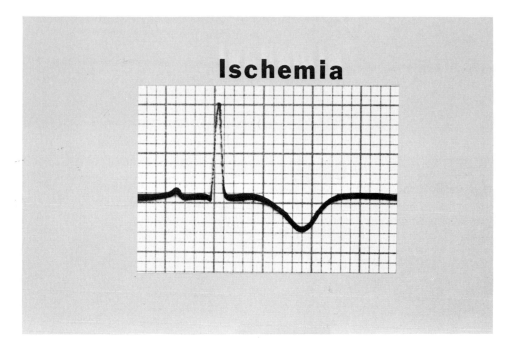

The typical Ischemia T wave is symmetrically inverted.

NOTE: With every EKG you should routinely check for T wave inversion. Since the chest leads are nearest the ventricles, T wave changes will be most pronounced in these leads. Always run down V_1–V_6 (as well as the limb leads) and check for T wave inversion* to see if there is diminished coronary blood flow.

The T wave of Ischemia is inverted and is
_____, that is the right and left sides   symmetrical
are mirror images.

*In adults flat (nonexistent) T waves or minimal T wave inversion may be a normal variant in any of the limb leads (frontal plane); however, any T wave inversion in leads V_2 through V_6 is considered pathological.

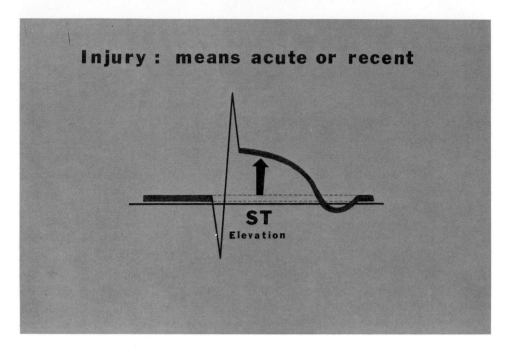

Injury : means acute or recent

ST
Elevation

Injury indicates the acuteness of an infarct, and the ST segment elevation denotes "injury."

NOTE: Acute means recent.

The ST segment is that section of baseline between the QRS complex and the _____ wave.

T

Elevation of the _____ segment signifies "injury." The ST segment may be only slightly elevated, or as much as ten or more millimeters above the baseline.

ST

The _____ of the ST segment gives us evidence that an infarct is acute.

elevation

ST Elevation

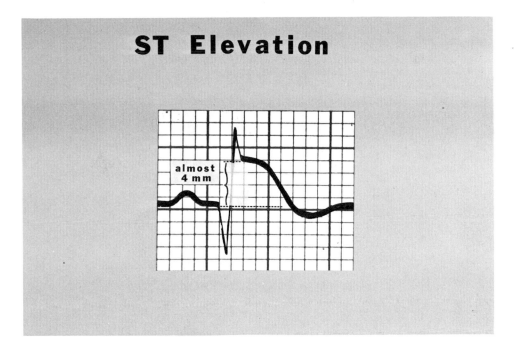

If there is ST elevation, this means that the infarction is acute; ST elevation alone may indicate a small infarction.

NOTE: If you have made the diagnosis of infarction, it is important to know whether the infarction just occurred and needs immediate treatment, or if the infarction is old— maybe years old.

The ST _____ rises above the baseline with an   segment
acute infarction and later returns to the level of the
baseline.

NOTE: If the ST segment is elevated without associated Q waves, this may represent "non-Q wave infarction," which is a small infarction that may herald an impending larger infarct. Significant ST changes require enzyme studies and close scrutiny.

NOTE: A ventricular aneurysm (the outward ballooning of the wall of a ventricle) may also cause ST elevation, but the ST segment in this case does *not* return to the baseline with time. Pericarditis may elevate the ST segment; however, the T wave is usually elevated off the baseline also (next page).

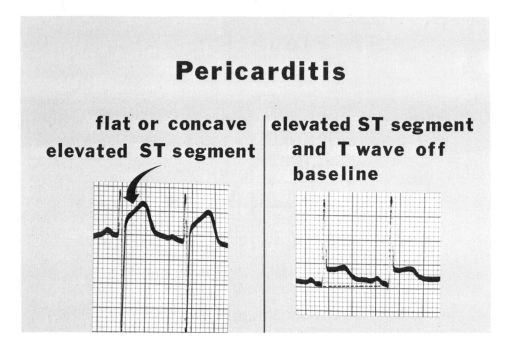

Pericarditis

flat or concave elevated ST segment | **elevated ST segment and T wave off baseline**

With *pericarditis* the ST segment is elevated, and it is usually flat or concave. The entire T wave may be elevated off the baseline.

NOTE: Pericarditis may be associated with infarction.

Pericarditis can _____ the ST segment. It will usually produce an elevated ST segment which is flat or slightly concave (middle sags downward); this resolves with time.

elevate

_____ seems to elevate the entire T wave off the baseline, that is, the baseline gradually angles back down (often including the P wave) all the way to the next QRS.

Pericarditis

NOTE: The characteristics shown in the left hand illustration are found in a lead in which the QRS is usually mainly negative (like the right chest leads). The pattern shown on the right hand illustration is seen in a lead where the QRS is mainly positive (like I or II).

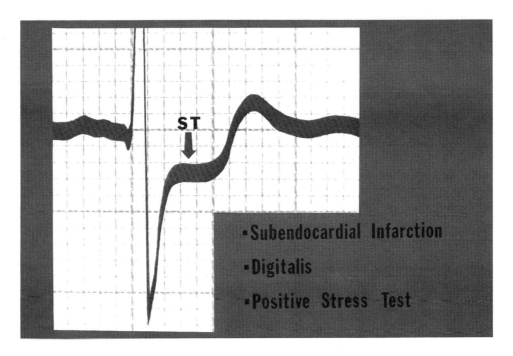

The ST segment may be depressed in certain conditions.

Digitalis may cause _____ of the ST   depression
segment.

> NOTE: During angina the ST segment is temporarily
> depressed, but this resolves when the anginal attack
> abates.

When a patient with suspected coronary Ischemia is
exercised, transient depression of the ___ segment may   ST
occur, confirming the diagnosis (Stress Test).

A _____ infarction—an infarct which   subendocardial
does not involve the full thickness of the left ventricle—will
depress the ST segment (see next page).

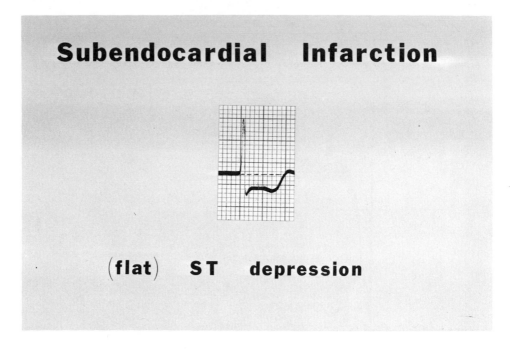

Subendocardial   Infarction

(flat)   S T   depression

Subendocardial infarction causes a classical flat (horizontal) depression of the ST segment; however, any significant ST depression should cause suspicion as to presence of subendocardial infarction.

Subendocardial infarction (it was originally called subendocardial injury) is identified by ST depression in which the ST _____ remains flat (horizontal or   segment downsloping).

NOTE: Subendocardial infarction, a type of "non-Q wave" infarction, involves only a small area of myocardium just below the endocardial lining. True myocardial infarctions usually involve the full thickness of (left) ventricular wall in the area which is affected. Even though subendocardial infarctions may involve only small areas of myocardial tissue, they should be treated much like a true M.I. Be cautious because subendocardial infarction is often considered a sign of impending myocardial infarction.

NOTE: Serum enzyme studies should be carried out with any acute ST depression (or elevation) which persists.

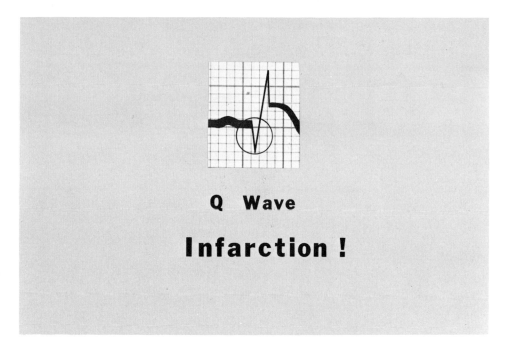

Q Wave

Infarction !

The Q wave makes the diagnosis of infarction.

The diagnosis of myocardial infarction is usually made by
the presence of Q _____.   waves

> NOTE: The Q wave is the first downward part of the QRS
> complex and is never preceded by anything in the complex.
> If there is any positive wave—even a tiny spike—in a
> QRS complex before the downward wave, we must call the
> downward wave an S wave (the upward part preceding it
> being an R wave).

Q waves are _____ in most of the leads in the tracing   absent
of a normal person.

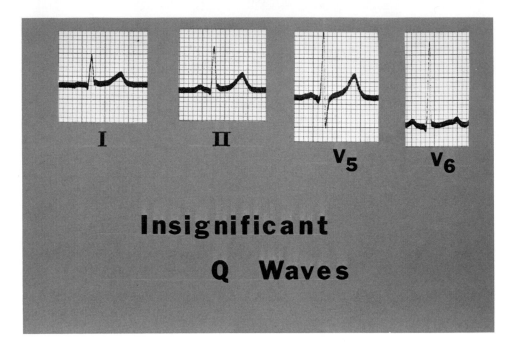

I II V₅ V₆

Insignificant Q Waves

Tiny insignificant Q waves may be seen normally in some leads.

Very small Q waves may be present _____ in certain leads. They usually represent normal septal depolarization.

normally

When these small Q waves are present, they are called _____ Q waves because they do not signify the presence of an infarction.

insignificant

Leads I, II, V₅, and V₆ commonly contain insignificant _____ waves.

Q

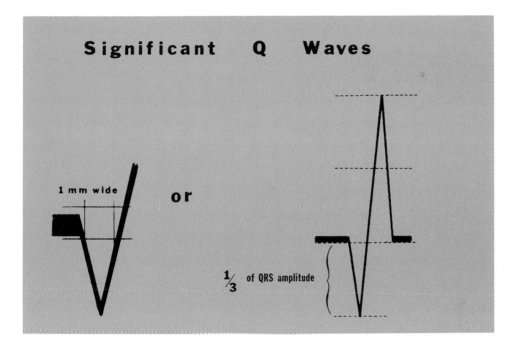

A *significant* Q wave is one small square wide (.04 sec.) or one-third of the amplitude of the entire QRS complex.

Significant _____ waves are indicative of pathology—namely the presence of an infarction.

Q

A significant Q wave is usually one small square (i.e., one millimeter) wide and is therefore _____ second in duration.

.04

Another helpful standard of a significant Q wave is when the Q wave is one-third the amplitude (height and depth) of the entire _____ complex.

QRS

NOTE: Currently, the width (duration) criteria for significant Q waves have taken precedence over those of depth (voltage). Some authors refer to significant Q waves as "pathological" Q waves for obvious reasons.

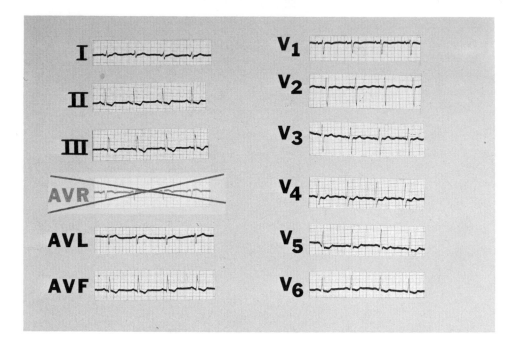

When looking at a tracing, note in which leads you can find significant Q waves. (Omit AVR.)

To check for infarction one should scan all the leads for the presence of _____ Q waves.   significant

> NOTE: Forget about lead AVR since this lead is positioned in such a way that data regarding Q waves is unreliable. Careful examination will reveal that lead AVR is like an upside-down lead II. So the large Q wave which is commonly seen in AVR is really the upside-down R wave from lead II. Even if you don't understand the logic behind AVR's phony Q's, don't check it for signs of infarction.

When checking a tracing, either on the long strip or mounted, write down those _____ in which you find   leads
significant Q waves, ST segment elevation (or depression), and inverted T waves . . . alone or in combination.

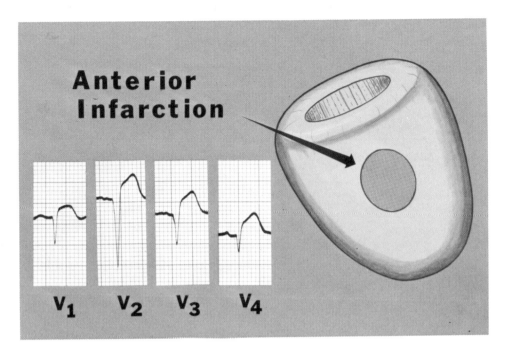

Anterior Infarction

V_1 V_2 V_3 V_4

Q waves in V_1, V_2, V_3, V_4 signify an *anterior* infarction. Is this one acute?

The presence of Q waves in leads V_1, V_2, V_3, or V_4 indicates an infarction in the anterior portion of the ＿＿＿＿ ventricle.

left

> NOTE: The anterior portion of the left ventricle includes part of the interventricular septum. Some cardiologists say that when Q waves appear in V_1 and V_2, these infarctions include the septum and are therefore often called "septal" infarctions. For all practical purposes, the presence of significant Q waves (remember V_5 and V_6 may have tiny normal Q's) in the chest leads means anterior infarction.

Anterior infarction may cause significant ＿＿ waves in any of the chest leads or just one chest lead. The chest leads are mainly *anteriorly* placed, and that's a good way to remember how to diagnose *anterior* infarction.

Q

> NOTE: Because of the ST elevation, this is an acute anterior infarction.

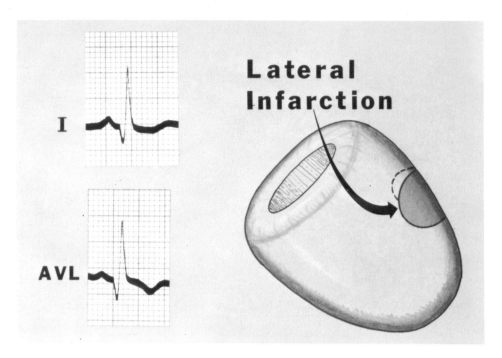

If there are **Q** waves in leads I and AVL, there is a *lateral* infarction.

A lateral infarction is one that has affected the portion of the _____ ventricle which is closest to the patient's *left* side.

left

When a lateral infarction occurs, it will cause **Q** _____ to appear in leads I and AVL. The one illustrated above is old.

waves

> NOTE: One might abbreviate Lateral Infarction as L.I. Just remember AVL for "Lateral" and "I" for Infarction (after all, Roman Numeral I is just a capital i). It's an easy way to recall the leads demonstrating lateral infarction.

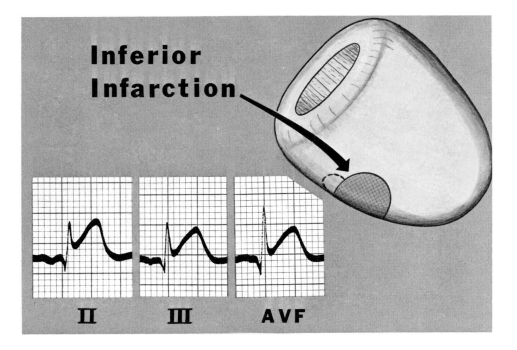

Inferior (diaphragmatic) infarction is designated by Q waves in II, III, and AVF.

The inferior wall of the heart rests upon the diaphragm so the term diaphragmatic infarction refers to an infarction in the inferior portion of the left _____.　　　　　ventricle

An _____ infarction is identified by significant　　　　inferior
Q waves in leads II, III, and AVF.

> NOTE: If I told you the way I remember the leads for inferior infarction, this book would be banned. An acute inferior infarction would probably be diagnosed by a person who notices significant Q waves in leads II, III, and AVF, and ST elevation in those leads. Is the one shown above acute?

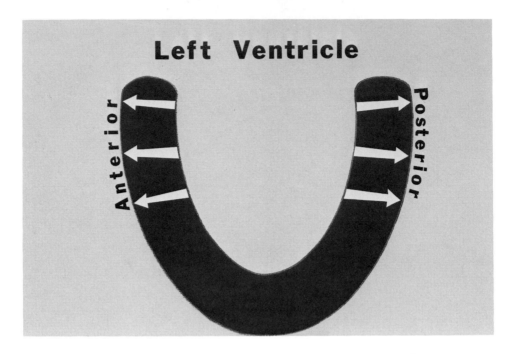

Note that the electrical activity of the anterior wall and posterior wall of the left ventricle is in opposite directions.

NOTE: Ventricular depolarization may be said to proceed from the *endocardium* (lining) to the *epicardium* (outside surface) of each ventricle.

Depolarization of the anterior wall of the left ventricle proceeds from the endocardium of the left ventricle anteriorly to the _____.

epicardium

Depolarization of the posterior wall of the _____ ventricle proceeds from the inner endocardium, which lines the left ventricle, through the full thickness of the ventricular wall to the outside ventricular surface (epicardium).

left

Vectors representing the depolarization of the anterior and posterior portions of the left ventricle point in _____ directions.

opposite

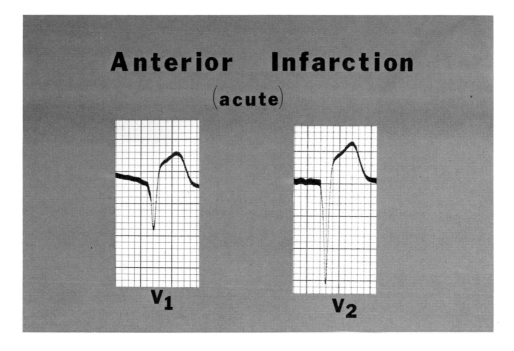

Anterior Infarction

(acute)

V₁   V₂

If an acute anterior infarction produces Q waves and ST elevation in V_1 and V_2, then a posterior infarction would appear the opposite.

An acute anterior infarction produces significant Q waves in the first few chest leads with ST _____ in the same leads.

elevation

Just considering V_1 and V_2 the appearance of significant Q waves and ST elevation would be indicative of acute _____ infarction.

anterior

NOTE: Acute posterior infarction of the left ventricle would produce the exact opposite to the pattern of acute anterior infarction, because the anterior and posterior walls of the left ventricle depolarize in opposite directions.

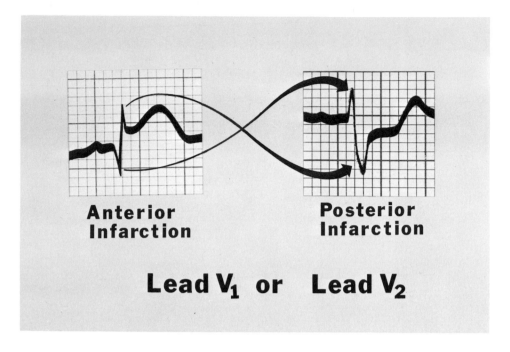

Anterior Infarction

Posterior Infarction

Lead V₁ or Lead V₂

In acute *posterior* infarction there is a large R wave (the opposite of a Q wave) in V_1 and V_2.

NOTE: In lead V_1, for instance, a Q wave turned upside-down would appear like an R wave (and as you will recall, R waves are usually very tiny in V_1).

A significant "Q wave" from an infarction in the posterior portion of the left _____ will cause a large R (positive deflection) wave in lead V_1.

ventricle

Suspect a true posterior infarction when you see a large _____ wave in V_1 or V_2, even though Right Ventricular Hypertrophy can cause them.

R

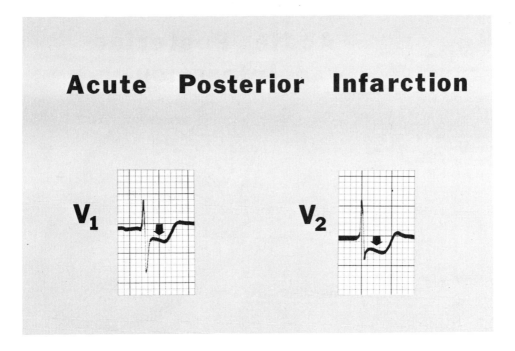

Acute Posterior Infarction

V_1 V_2

In acute posterior infarction, there will also be ST depression (opposite of the "usual" elevation) in V_1 or V_2.

An acute anterior infarction will cause Q waves in the chest leads and the ST segments will be _____.   elevated

NOTE: Since the posterior wall of the left ventricle depolarizes in a direction opposite to that of the anterior wall, an acute infarct to the posterior wall will cause ST *DEPRESSION* in V_1 or V_2.

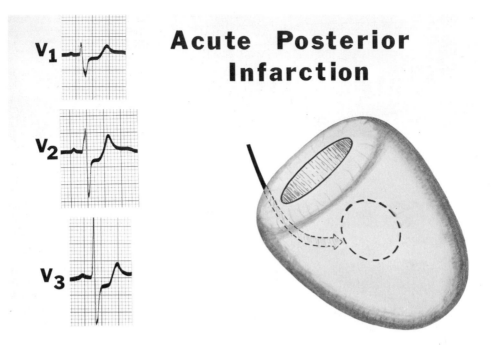

Acute Posterior Infarction

In summary, acute posterior infarction is characterized by a large R wave and ST depression in V_1, V_2 (and/or V_3).

NOTE: Always be suspicious of ST segment depression in the right chest leads—it could indicate a true posterior (acute) infarction. (If you do not recall those things which can cause ST depression, look back at page 223). The diagnosis (see page 224) of an *anterior subendocardial infarction* (because of depressed ST segments in chest leads) should be made with extreme caution, because this may really represent an acute true posterior infarct.

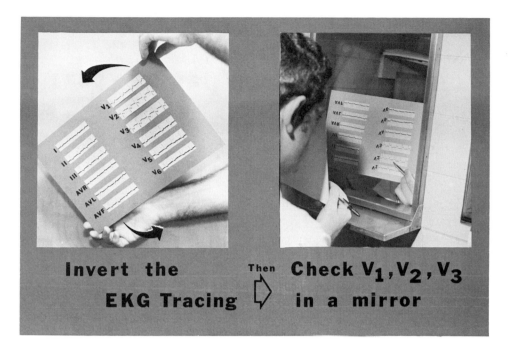

Invert the EKG Tracing Then ⇨ **Check V₁, V₂, V₃ in a mirror**

If an acute posterior infarction is suspected (large R and ST depression in V_1 or V_2), try the "mirror test."

NOTE: If a posterior infarction is suspected by tall R waves and ST depression in V_1 or V_2, try the mirror test:

First, turn the entire tracing upside-down. Then, look at V_1 and V_2 in a mirror and you should see the classical signs of acute infarction, i.e., a big Q wave and ST elevation. Try this maneuver with the illustration on the previous page. It is an easy maneuver to perform, if you can keep from looking at yourself in the mirror.

This test consists of two maneuvers, namely inverting the tracing and looking at the inverted V_1 and V_2 in a
_____.

mirror

Always Check V_1 and V_2 for:

1. ST elevation and Q waves (Anterior Infarct)

2. ST depression and large R waves (Posterior Infarct)

Although posterior infarctions are very severe, they are easy to overlook.

When making your routine reading of an EKG, pay special attention to leads V_1 and _____ while looking for signs of infarction.

V_2

NOTE: ST changes in leads V_1 and V_2 are always significant and important, both depression *and* elevation.

Check for Q waves in V_1 and V_2 and also observe the height of the _____ waves.

R

NOTE: And remember how important T wave inversion can be in all leads.

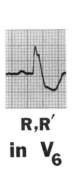

R,R′

in V₆

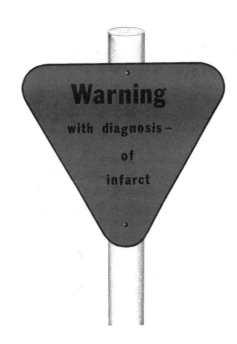

The EKG diagnosis of infarction is generally not valid in the presence of Left Bundle Branch Block.

In Left Bundle Block, the left ventricle (which generally is the only chamber to infarct) depolarizes after the _____ ventricle.

right

So any Q wave originating from the left ventricle could not appear at the beginning of the QRS _____ (with Left B.B.B.) and would fall somewhere in the middle of the QRS complex. Thus it would be difficult to identify significant Q's in this case.

complex

> NOTE: One special exception is possible. The right and left ventricle share the interventricular septum in common. So an infarct in the septal area would be shared by the right ventricle which depolarizes first in Left B.B.B. This would produce Q waves at the beginning of the wide QRS. Therefore even in the presence of the Left B.B.B., Q waves in the chest leads might make one suspect (but not confirm) septal (anterior) infarction.

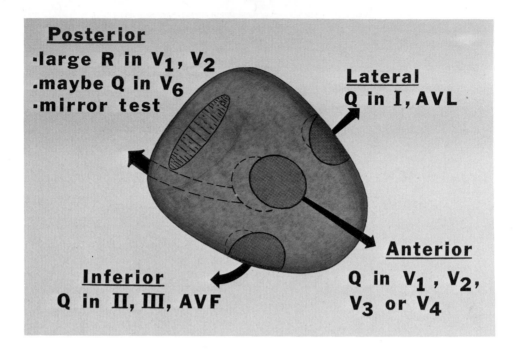

Posterior
- large R in V$_1$, V$_2$
- maybe Q in V$_6$
- mirror test

Lateral
Q in I, AVL

Anterior
Q in V$_1$, V$_2$,
V$_3$ or V$_4$

Inferior
Q in II, III, AVF

Locating an infarct is important because the prognosis depends on the location of the infarction.

There are _____ general locations within the left ventricle where infarctions commonly occur.

four

NOTE: More than one area in the left ventricle may infarct. One area may be very old and one very recent, so correlate the ST elevation with the appropriate leads for the location of an infarct. If ST elevation is present in leads *without* Q waves, "non-Q wave" infarction must be ruled out.

Be careful about diagnosing an infarction in the presence of a _____ Bundle Branch Block.

Left

NOTE: Isolated areas of Ischemia (T inversion) or ST elevation (non-Q wave infarction) can also be "located" using the same location criteria.

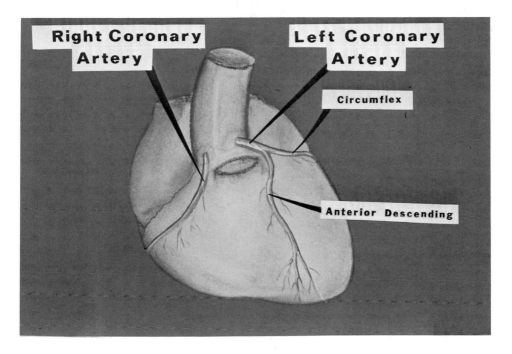

Locating infarctions is a common practice, but with a little anatomical knowledge of the heart's coronary blood supply,* we can make a far more sophisticated diagnosis.

There are _____ coronary arteries which provide the heart with a nutrient supply of oxygenated blood.   two

The Left coronary artery has two major branches; they are the Circumflex branch and the Anterior _____ branch.   Descending

The _____ coronary artery curves around the right ventricle.   Right

*The pulmonary artery has been surgically removed from this illustration to show the origin of the coronary arteries at the base of the aorta.

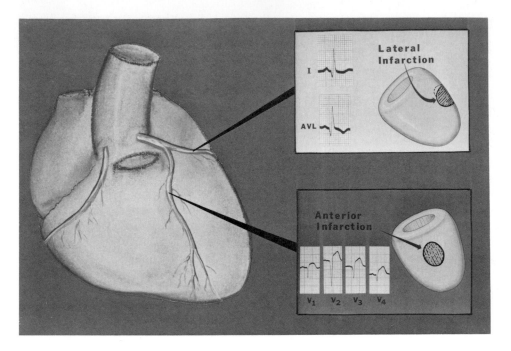

A lateral infarction is caused by an occlusion of the Circumflex branch of the Left coronary artery. An anterior infarction is due to an occlusion of the Anterior Descending branch of the Left coronary artery.

The Circumflex branch of the Left coronary artery distributes blood to the _____ portion of left ventricle.   lateral

The Anterior Descending branch of the left coronary artery supplies the _____ part of the left ventricle with blood.   anterior

The Circumflex and the Anterior Descending are the two main branches of the _____ coronary artery.   Left

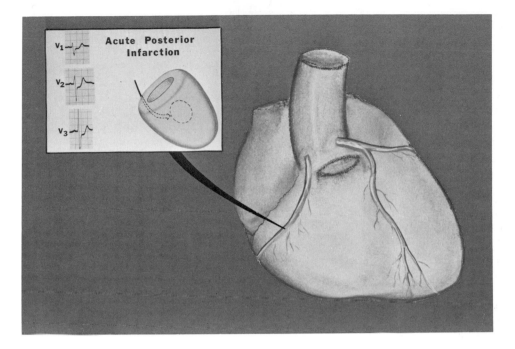

True posterior infarctions are generally due to an occlusion of the Right coronary artery or one of its smaller branches.

The _____ coronary artery swings around behind the right ventricle to supply the posterior portion of the left ventricle.

Right

A posterior infarction is caused by an occlusion of a branch of the Right _____ artery.

coronary

NOTE: For a long time the Right coronary artery was considered to play only a minor role in the blood supply of the heart. The sophisticated techniques of coronary angiography have shown that the Right coronary artery usually provides the local blood supply to the SA Node, AV Node, and the (AV) Bundle of His. It is no wonder that acute posterior infarctions are often associated with dangerous arrhythmias. Wise cardiologists have great concern and respect for the posterior M.I.

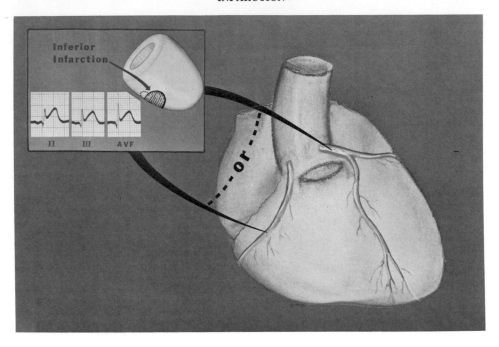

The *base* of the left ventricle obtains its blood supply from either the right or the left coronary branches, depending on which artery is *dominant*.

Inferior (or "diaphragmatic") infarctions are caused by an
_____ of either the Right or Left coronary   occlusion
artery branches.

So the diagnosis of inferior _____ does not   infarction
identify the artery branch which is occluded, unless you
have a previous coronary angiogram (an x-ray highlighting
the coronary arteries) to show which artery has supplied the
inferior portion of the heart (in that particular patient).

> NOTE: Radiologists define Left or Right coronary
> "dominance" as denoting which artery renders the greatest
> portion of blood supply to the base of the left ventricle in a
> given patient. For instance, if the coronary angiogram of a
> patient demonstrates that his left coronary artery renders
> most of the blood supply to the base of the left ventricle,
> there is basal "dominance" of the left coronary artery in
> that patient.

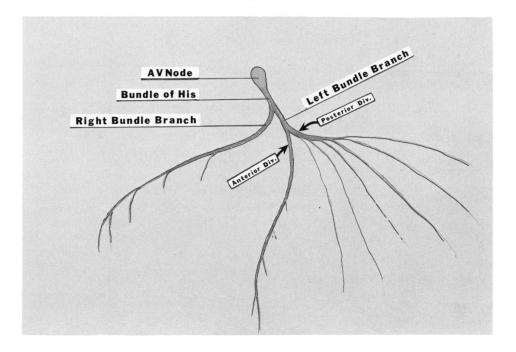

Hemiblocks are presented in this section (Infarction) because they are commonly associated with infarction and a resultant diminished blood supply to the Bundle Branch conduction system.

The hemiblocks are blocks of the anterior or posterior division of the _____ Bundle Branch.

Left

Hemiblocks are commonly (but not always) due to loss of blood supply to either the Anterior or _____ division of the Left Bundle Branch.

Posterior

NOTE: The Right Bundle Branch does not have significant, recognizable divisions of either clinical or electrocardiographic importance (yet).

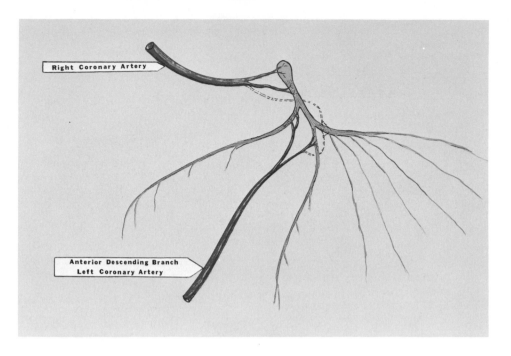

Right Coronary Artery

Anterior Descending Branch
Left Coronary Artery

To understand hemiblocks, one must understand the blood supply to the AV Node and the ventricular conduction system.

The Right coronary artery usually renders a blood supply* to the AV Node, Bundle of His, and a variable twig to the Posterior division of the Left _____ Branch.

Bundle

The Left coronary artery also sends a variable twig of _____ supply to the Posterior division of the Left Bundle Branch.

blood

A total occlusion of the Anterior Descending branch of the left coronary artery may cause a subsequent Right Bundle Branch _____ and also an Anterior Hemiblock.

Block

NOTE: The key to understanding Hemiblocks is to keep in mind that an infarction may be due to an occlusion of a vessel at any of numerous locations, and therefore may cause a variety of blocks of the Bundle Branch system, i.e., single blocks of one bundle or division, or combinations of these blocks sparing one or more branches. An occlusion which is not quite complete may cause an *intermittent* block.

*Let's not forget that the SA Node is usually dependent on the right coronary artery.

Anterior Hemiblock

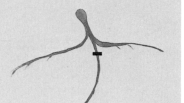

- L.A.D. - usually assoc. with an M.I. (or other heart disease)

- QRS slightly widened (.10 to .12)

- $Q_1 S_3$

Anterior Hemiblock refers to a block of the anterior division of the Left Bundle Branch and the above criteria are used in the diagnosis.

The slight delay of conduction to the antero-lateral and superior area of the left ventricle causes (late) unopposed depolarization upward to the left recognized as Left _____ Deviation. Acute L.A.D. is generally what makes one suspect Anterior Hemiblock.

Axis

With pure Anterior Hemiblock, the QRS is widened only .10 to .12 sec., but association with other blocks of the _____ Branch system may widen the QRS more.

Bundle

Anterior Hemiblock is usually verified by a Q in I and a wide and/or deep _____ in III ($Q_1 S_3$).

S

> NOTE: Previous tracings are essential in making Anterior (or any) Hemiblock diagnosis. You *must* always rule out pre-existing sources of Left Axis Deviation, e.g., Left Ventricular Hypertrophy, Horizontal Heart, or Inferior Infarction.

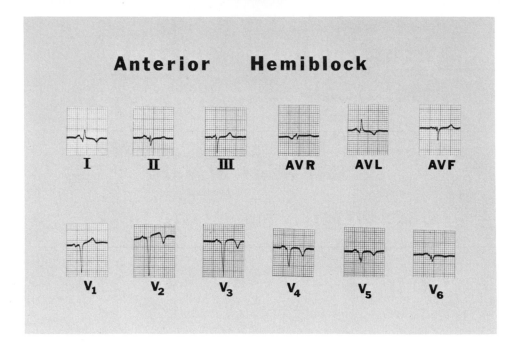

An occlusion of the Anterior Descending coronary artery produces an Anterior Infarction, and about one-half of these patients develop Anterior Hemiblock.

Anterior Hemiblock describes a block of the Anterior Division of the Left Bundle Branch causing a delay in depolarization to that (antero-lateral, and superior) area of the left _____, to produce Left Axis Deviation.

ventricle

An occlusion of the *Anterior* Descending coronary artery will produce an *Anterior* Infarction which often causes *Anterior* _____ . (that's easy to remember).

Hemiblock

If a patient with an acute Anterior Infarction has an Axis change from normal to −60°, suspect Anterior _____ (and look for Q_1S_3).

Hemiblock

But if a patient with an Inferior Infarction develops Left Axis Deviation, beware! Inferior Infarction can cause L.A.D., so _____ Hemiblock is not the prime suspect.

Anterior

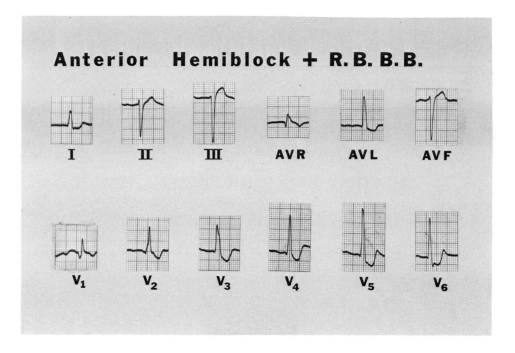

Anterior Hemiblock + R.B.B.B.

An infarction of the anterior wall of the left ventricle (due to occlusion of the Anterior Descending branch of the left coronary artery) may cause Anterior Hemiblock (and R.B.B.B.).

NOTE: Don't forget that the Anterior Descending Artery also renders blood supply to the Right Bundle Branch, so Anterior Infarction may have an assorted R.B.B.B. depending on the level of occlusion.

With Right Bundle Branch Block the Mean QRS Vector is within the normal range or shows minimal Right Axis _____ .   Deviation

However, when a patient develops a Right Bundle Branch Block with Left Axis Deviation as well, this is probably due to Anterior Hemiblock, particularly if there is an acute Anterior _____ .   Infarction

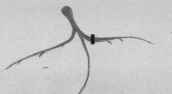

Posterior Hemiblock

· **R.A.D.** - **usually assoc. with an M.I.**
  (**or other heart disease**)

· **Normal or slightly widened QRS**

· **S_1Q_3**

Pure isolated *Posterior Hemiblock* is rare because the posterior division is short, thick, and commonly has a dual blood supply.

An inferior infarction may destroy the blood supply to the Posterior division of the Left Bundle _____.

Branch

Posterior Hemiblocks cause _____ Axis Deviation due to the late, unopposed depolarization forces toward the right.

Right

Look for a deep or unusually wide S in I and Q in III known as S_1Q_3 when _____ Hemiblock is suspected.

Posterior

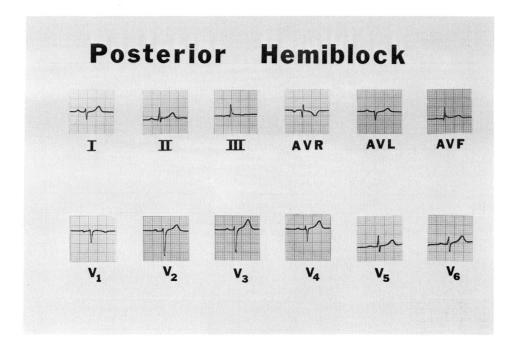

Posterior Hemiblock is always to be respected, and all Inferior Infarctions should be scrutinized to rule it out.

A lateral infarction, either recent or old, may produce Right Axis _____ which can be confused with Posterior Hemiblock. It is said that in the presence of lateral M.I., the EKG diagnosis of Posterior Hemiblock is equivocal.

Deviation

Make certain that by history and previous EKG's, chronic _____ Axis Deviation due to slender body build, Right Ventricular Hypertrophy, and pulmonary disease, etc., is ruled out.

Right

Posterior _____ is serious, and when in association with Right Bundle Branch Block, they are considered very dangerous because of the predisposition of progression into AV Blocks.

Hemiblock

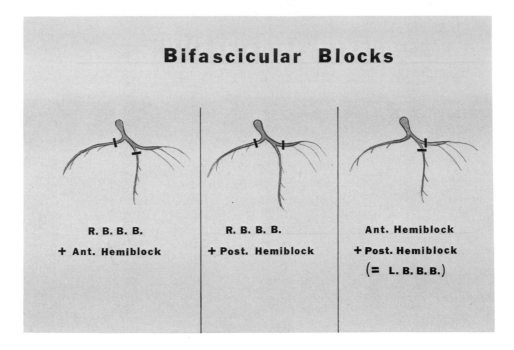

Bifascicular Blocks

R. B. B. B.
+ Ant. Hemiblock

R. B. B. B.
+ Post. Hemiblock

Ant. Hemiblock
+ Post. Hemiblock
(= L. B. B.B.)

The word fascicle means bundle, so any main division of the ventricular conduction system is a fascicle.

NOTE: For many years "Bundle" referred to either the Right or Left Bundle Branch. When referring to combinations of blocks (e.g., Hemiblock + Bundle Branch Block) we use the word "fascicular" block to imply a Bundle Branch Block and a Hemiblock (fascicle means bundle literally).

NOTE: *Bi*fascicular block means *two* fascicles are blocked. Because Anterior Hemiblock plus Posterior Hemiblock is generally indistinguishable from Left Bundle Branch Block, Bifascicular Block generally refers to Right Bundle Branch Block together with a block of either the Anterior Division or the Posterior Division of the Left Bundle Branch.

NOTE: Any block location may be *intermittent,* so the EKG signs may only appear from time to time (next page).

Intermittent Blocks
...with at least one normal, non-blocked fascicle

Intermittent block of one fascicle: continuous EKG pattern of normal with intermittent signs of block.

Intermittent block of two fascicles: intermittent EKG signs of both blocks.

Intermittent block:
one intermittent + one permanent block
... continuous EKG pattern of one block
and intermittent signs of another block.

Fortunately, combinations of [fascicular] blocks are often *intermittent,* so that when in combination with other blocks they are more easily recognized and treated.

A patient with a block of one or more fascicles may have an associated intermittent _____ of another fascicle producing intermittent (or occasional) signs of block of another fascicle.

block

A patient may have a permanent fascicular block and an intermittent block in one or more of the other _____.

fascicles

Intermittent block may exist in more than one fascicle in the same patient at once, producing intermittent _____ signs (as varying Axis).

EKG

> NOTE: Like a faulty light bulb which occasionally (intermittently) does not light, fascicles may suffer intermittent block. And like a faulty, flickering light bulb which eventually blows out, intermittent fascicular blocks often warn of impending *permanent* block of that fascicle. When permanent blocks of other fascicles already exist, intermittent fascicular block is a warning to the clinician that an artificial pacemaker may be necessary (see next page). That is why the first printed word in this page is "Fortunately."

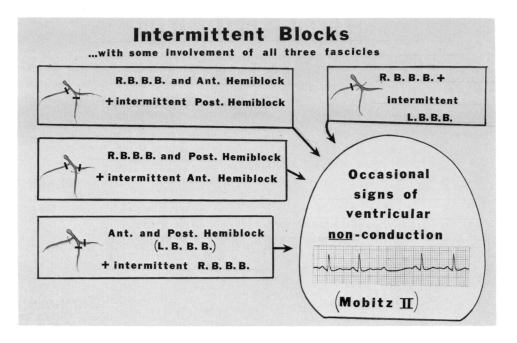

Intermittent Blocks
...with some involvement of all three fascicles

R.B.B.B. and Ant. Hemiblock
+intermittent Post. Hemiblock

R.B.B.B. + intermittent L.B.B.B.

R.B.B.B. and Post. Hemiblock
+ intermittent Ant. Hemiblock

Ant. and Post. Hemiblock (L.B.B.B.)
+ intermittent R.B.B.B.

Occasional signs of ventricular **non**-conduction

(Mobitz II)

Considering the three pathways of ventricular depolarization, it becomes apparent that one [fascicle] must remain open at least intermittently to provide ventricular conduction.

*Tri*fascicular blocks are diagnosed only when one or more of the fascicular _____ is intermittent.

blocks

The diagnosis of "Bilateral" (left and right) Bundle _____ Block similarly is made only if the block is intermittent somewhere in one or both of the Bundles.

Branch

Complete, permanent Trifascicular block or Bilateral Bundle Branch Block is indistinguishable from complete (3°) AV _____.

Block

NOTE: If all fascicles are permanently blocked except one which is intermittently blocked, a Mobitz II type pattern (i.e., occasional nonconduction to ventricles or runs of 2:1 [or worse] AV conduction) will emerge. So the sudden appearance of Mobitz II patterns should alert you to the potential need for an External Non-invasive Pacemaker, and you should consider the eventual need for permanent pacemaker implantation. Review and understand the illustrations.

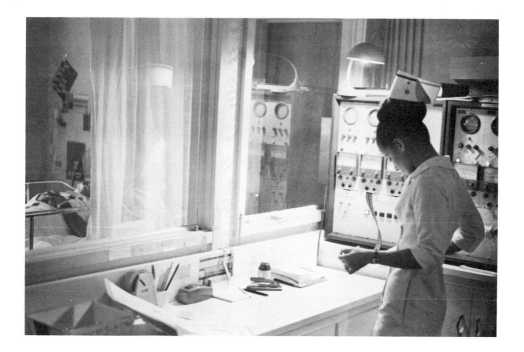

In most hospitals, patients with acute myocardial infarctions are placed in coronary care units and monitored continuously; indeed, all patients with suspected infarctions are usually placed in such units.

NOTE: Just as the preferred treatment of various arrhythmias changes with the times, so the attitudes toward indications for implantation of artificial pacemakers are constantly changing relative to AV Blocks, Bundle Branch and fascicular blocks, intermittent blocks, etc. Therefore, it is essential that you keep up with the current medical literature.

The subject of severity of infarction relative to its position in the left _____ is very controversial, so   ventricle each one of us must be well read on the subject to make his or her own decisions.

NOTE: Infarctions may "extend" or progressively involve a larger area of the left ventricle. Obviously, extension of acute infarction carries a less favorable prognosis than the original infarct.

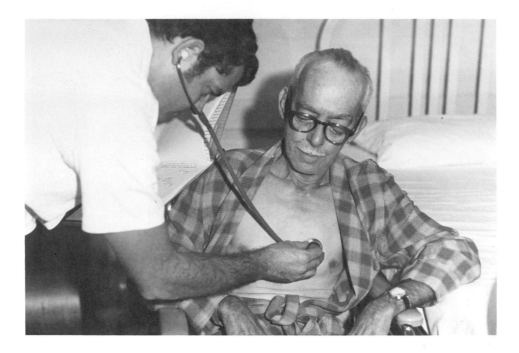

Remember that the history and clinical diagnosis are still the most important standards in the determination of acute infarction.

The EKG has been called "only an aid" in the diagnosis of myocardial _____ even though it probably gives more specific information than any other parameter.

infarction

There is no substitute for taking and evaluating a thorough _____.

history

The laboratory also gives us many ways to evaluate the status of the patient, but careful _____ interpretation is essential.

EKG

NOTE: The electrocardiogram is a useful diagnostic tool, but its value increases multifold when it is compared to a patient's previous tracings. Always attempt to obtain a patient's previous EKG's for comparison, because electrocardiograms, like X-rays, become much more valuable when we can ascertain whether the pathology is recent or old. Incidentally, is this a photo of Dr. Paul Dudley White, and who is his examining physician?

NOTE: Review Infarction by turning to the **P**ersonal **Q**uick **R**eference **S**heets at the end of this book on pages 288 and 289, and note your simplified methodology (page 280).

Miscellaneous Effects

Pulmonary

Electrolytes

Medications

Artificial Pacemakers

Heart Transplants

The above effects, which are common to, but not diagnostic of, certain conditions, can produce recognizable changes in the EKG.

NOTE: These following effects may be recognized by a characteristic appearance on electrocardiogram. For most of the conditions mentioned in this section, these electrocardiographic signs merely make one aware of existing conditions, certain pathology, or drug or electrolyte effects. In most instances, review of the medical history, detailed physical exam, or diagnostic tests will be necessary to confirm your suspicion. Rarely is a diagnosis made entirely on the existence of any of the following EKG findings.

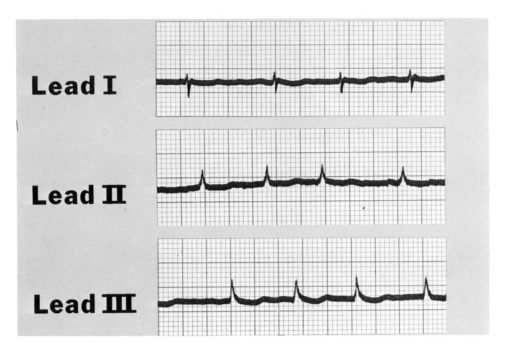

Emphysema usually produces low voltage in all leads, and there is often Right Axis Deviation.

Severe _____ commonly produces QRS   emphysema
complexes of small amplitude in all leads.* Indeed, this
pulmonary disease diminishes the voltage of all waves in all
leads.

With pulmonary emphysema the right ventricle is working
against resistance; this may cause _____ Axis   Right
Deviation.

The Right Axis Deviation is usually due to Right
Ventricular Hypertrophy. We can diagnose Right Axis
Deviation by simply noting that the _____ in lead I is   QRS
mainly negative.

*Low voltage in all leads is also seen with hypothyroidism and chronic constrictive pericarditis.

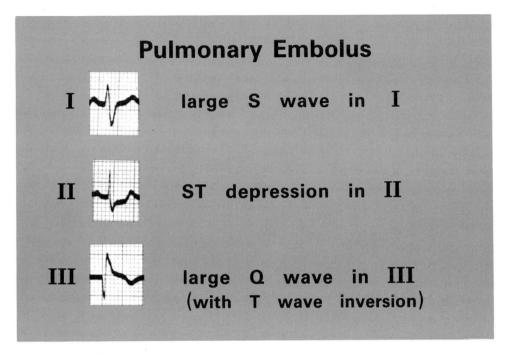

Pulmonary Embolus

I   large S wave in I

II   ST depression in II

III   large Q wave in III
(with T wave inversion)

With *Pulmonary Embolus* we commonly see a large S wave in lead I, and a Q wave and an inverted T wave in lead III ($S_1Q_3L_3$)*.

$S_1Q_3L_3$ syndrome characterizes acute cor pulmonale as a result of pulmonary embolus. It is called $S_1Q_3L_3$ because of the large S wave in lead I, and there is a Q wave and an inverted T wave in lead _____.   III

NOTE: Observe the tendency toward Right Axis Deviation (lead I).

There is also usually ST _____ in lead II.   depression

*Don't be confused by the inversion of the T wave in the printed text. It is an excellent memory tool, even if the publisher dislikes it.

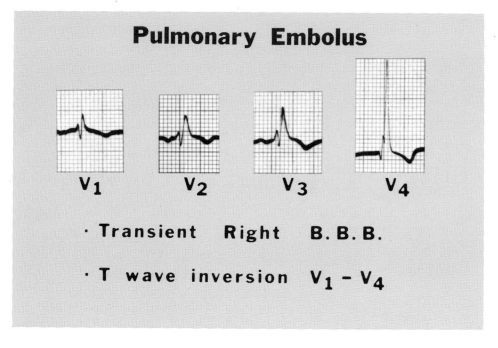

Pulmonary Embolus

V_1 V_2 V_3 V_4

· Transient Right B.B.B.

· T wave inversion $V_1 - V_4$

Also with Pulmonary Embolus there is commonly T wave inversion in V_1 through V_4. There is often transient Right Bundle Branch Block.

_____ wave inversion in the chest leads, particularly lead V_1 T
through V_4 is a very important diagnostic sign of
pulmonary embolus.

Pulmonary _____ may cause Right Bundle   Embolus
Branch Block. This block usually subsides after the patient
improves.

We can recognize the presence of Right Bundle Branch
Block by the R,R' in the _____ chest leads.   right

     NOTE: Occasionally the Right B.B.B. may be "incomplete"
(QRS complex of normal width, but R,R' is present).

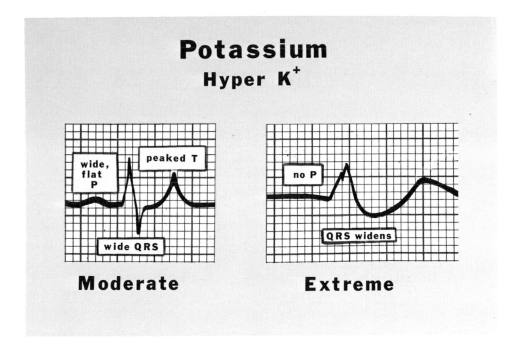

Potassium
Hyper K⁺

Moderate — wide, flat P; peaked T; wide QRS

Extreme — no P; QRS widens

With *elevated serum potassium* the P wave flattens down, the QRS complex widens, and the T wave becomes peaked.

With an elevated serum potassium, the T wave becomes
_____.

peaked

The P wave will flatten down until it is difficult to find
in extreme _____.

hyperkalemia

When a patient has an elevated potassium, ventricular
depolarization takes longer, and the QRS complex
subsequently _____.

widens

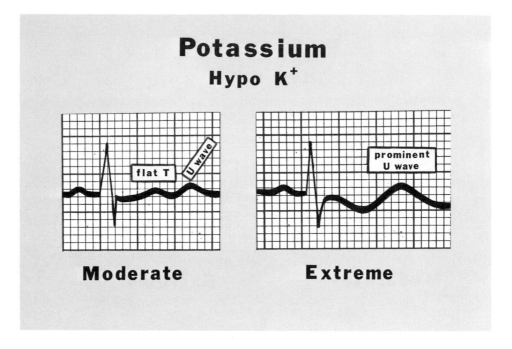

Potassium
Hypo K$^+$

Moderate   **Extreme**

As the serum potassium drops below normal, the T wave becomes flat (or inverted) and there is a U wave.

With low serum potassium, the T wave becomes flat as the _____ drops. As the potassium level becomes lower, the T wave may become inverted.

potassium

> NOTE: I always think of the T wave as a tent housing potassium ions. As the potassium ions fall below normal, the T wave flattens down. Conversely, increased potassium ions will peak the T wave upward.

With hypokalemia a _____ wave appears. This wave becomes more prominent as the loss of potassium becomes more severe.

U

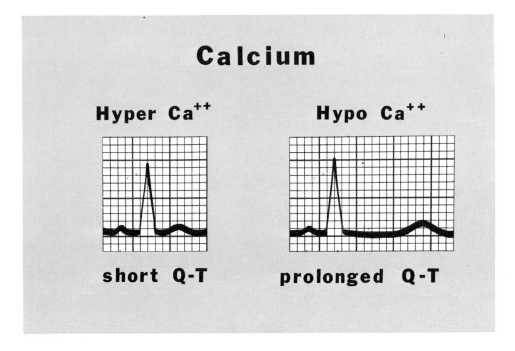

With *hypercalcemia* the Q-T interval shortens, but with *hypocalcemia* the Q-T interval becomes prolonged.

Hypocalcemia will usually _____ the Q-T interval.

prolong

NOTE: The Q-T interval is measured from the beginning of the QRS complex to the *end* of the T wave.

Increased serum Calcium apparently enhances rapid ventricular repolarization (after depolarization). This produces a short _____ interval.

Q-T

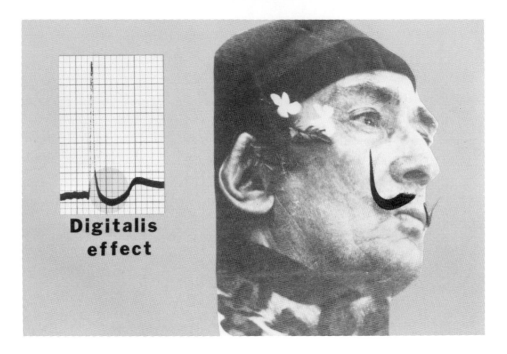

Digitalis effect

Digitalis causes gradual downward sloping of the ST segment to give it the appearance of Salvador Dali's mustache.

Digitalis produces a unique gradual down-sloping of the _____ segment, this is the classical "digitalis effect."

ST

> NOTE: Find a lead with no demonstrable S wave to identify this classic pattern. The downward portion of the R wave gradually becomes thicker as it approaches the baseline. The downward limb of the R wave has a gentle curving, downward slope as it blends into the baseline. Note that the ST segment is slightly depressed as it sags downward. This pattern can be demonstrated on the EKG's of most digitalized patients.*

*Digitalis tends to slow the heart rate and can cause Sinus Bradycardia even with therapeutic levels.

Excess Digitalis

· **S A Block**

· **P. A. T. with Block**

· **A V Blocks**

· **Tachycardia with A V dissociation**

Excess digitalis tends to cause AV Blocks of many varieties, and may cause Sinus (SA) Block.

Digitalis in _____ may cause Sinus (SA) Block.

excess

Digitalis in excess will retard or block conduction of the depolarization stimulus through the AV _____.

Node

_____ digitalis may cause various types of AV Block and even tachycardia associated with AV block.

Excess

NOTE: Always be aware of the fact that digitalis excess is exaggerated by low serum potassium.

Digitalis Toxicity

- **P.V.C. 's**
- **Bigeminy, Trigeminy, etc.**
- **Ventricular Tachycardia**
- **Ventricular Fibrillation**
- **Atrial Fibrillation**

Digitalis in toxic amounts will stimulate ectopic foci to discharge and cause subsequent arrhythmias.

Digitalis in _____ amounts can produce irritable   toxic
ectopic foci, particularly in the ventricles.

Dangerous arrhythmias may arise from ventricular ectopic
_____ discharging often or even firing repetitively at a   foci
tachycardia rate.

> NOTE: Digitalis preparations have been the physician's friend in treating cardiac failure since the thirteenth century. It must be respected, however, because in toxic amounts it can cause deadly arrhythmias.

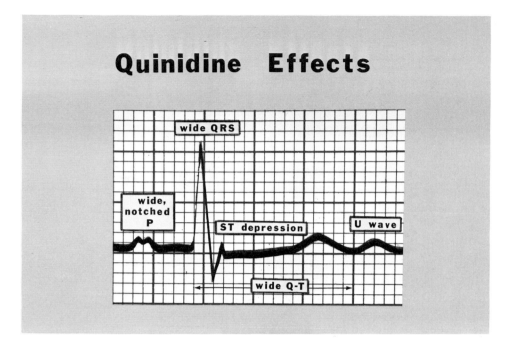

Quinidine causes notching of a widened P wave as well as widening of the QRS complex. There is often ST depression, a prolonged Q-T, and U waves.

NOTE: Quinidine retards electrical conduction through the myocardium. Most of the effects of quinidine noted on EKG are related to a slowing of the speed of depolarization and repolarization.

Quinidine causes a wide, notched _____ wave on EKG and also widens the QRS complex.

P

Quinidine can prolong the _____ interval, and depress the ST segment. Look for U waves.

Q-T

Quinidine Toxicity

Torsades de Pointes

Torsades de Pointes is considered a sign of Quinidine toxicity.

Torsades de Pointes is a ventricular tachycardia
(rate 200–250/min.) which originates in a
_____ focus and usually is a brief self-   ventricular
resolving episode, but it may be dangerous.

    NOTE: The amplitude of the sine-wave-like complexes
gradually increases then gradually decreases causing a
classical spindle shaped progression of waves.

Although other causes of Q-T interval widening may be
implicated, _____ toxicity is probably the   quinidine
most common cause.

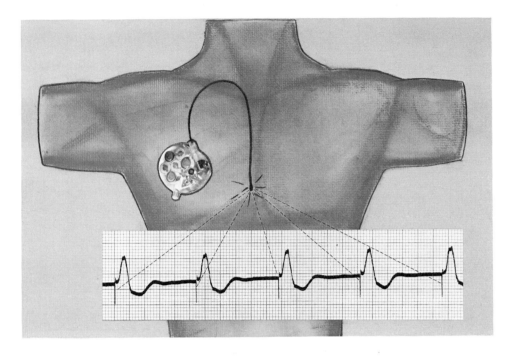

The artificial (battery operated) pacemaker produces regular electrical stimuli (spikes). Immediately after each spike we expect to see a ventricular response; however, there are many types which also stimulate the atria.

NOTE: Artificial pacemakers are surgically implanted in symptomatic patients with third degree (complete) AV Block.* In 3° (complete) Block, the ventricular rate may be so slow (20–40/min.) that a battery operated pacemaker is needed to keep the heart pumping at a normal rate. The battery portion is implanted under the skin, and the wire lead is either passed through the venous system into the right ventricle ("transvenous"), or (rarely) an electrode is sewn to the outside of the left ventricle wall ("epicardial").

The pacemaker emits an _____ impulse regularly, producing a small ventricle spike on EKG (more complex varieties are also in use).

electrical

We expect each impulse to "capture" (i.e., depolarize) the ventricles. Because this artificial ventricular depolarization is "ectopic" each ventricular response will look like a _____.

P.V.C.

*Currently, signs of "impending" complete block (see pages 253, 254) are a strong indication for pacemaker implantations.

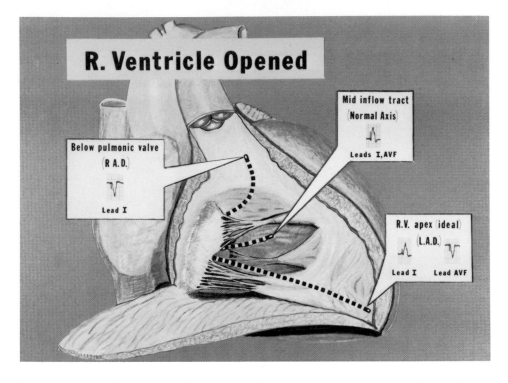

Right Ventricular pacemakers are the most common type; the catheter-electrode tip is within the cavity of the right ventricle.

NOTE: The most ideal location for a Right Ventricular (transvenous) pacemaker is to have the catheter-electrode tip at the apex of the right ventricular cavity. The resultant QRS has a L.B.B.B. pattern with Left Axis Deviation.

When a paced QRS shows a L.B.B.B. _____ with a normal axis, the catheter-electrode tip is in the Right Ventricular mid-inflow tract.

pattern

But if one sees a paced QRS with a L.B.B.B. pattern and Right Axis Deviation, the _____-electrode tip is just below the pulmonic valves.

catheter

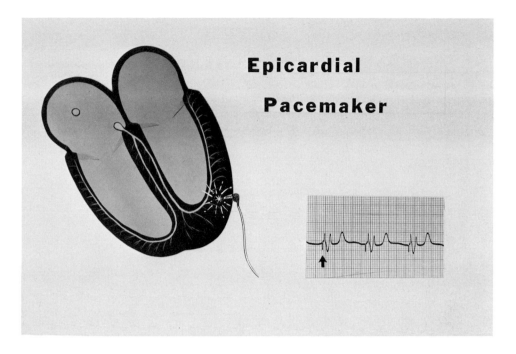

The electrode tip of an Epicardial Pacemaker is surgically attached to the outer surface of the left ventricle.

The electrode tip of an epicardial pacemaker is located on the epicardial surface of the left _____, so the left ventricle depolarizes before the right, and

ventricle

. . . this produces a QRS with a Right Bundle _____ Block pattern.

Branch

Epicardial pacemakers produce a QRS with a _____ Bundle Branch Block pattern and usually Right Axis Deviation as well. They are not used commonly.

Right

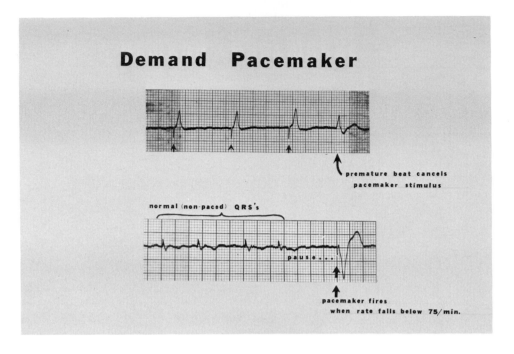

The "demand" pacemaker has sensing ability, a ready pacemaker stimulus, and a "brain" to determine when to pace and when to stop.

The demand pacemaker will fire on "demand" when it senses a _____ in rate below a predetermined level.

decrease

. . . and should the rate return (to normal), the demand _____ will sense the normal rhythm and shut itself off so it will not compete with the normal rhythm.

pacemaker

The _____ pacemaker can sense a P.V.C. so that the next pacemaker stimulus will "reset" in step with the P.V.C., that is, it begins after an interval (i.e., after the P.V.C.) which is similar to the usual interval between paced beats.

demand

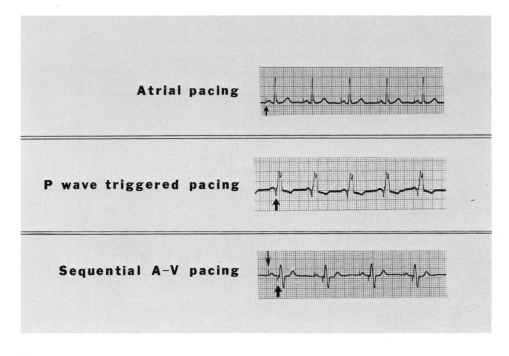

These are a few examples of some of the many types of artificial pacemakers.

In atrial pacing, the pacemaker stimulates the _____ and conduction proceeds normally in the remainder of each cycle.

atria

However, in P wave triggered pacing, the pacemaker unit senses the P wave, and then fires a (ventricular) _____ shortly thereafter. (This is also called "atrial synchronous" pacing).

stimulus

In sequential A-V pacing, the pacemaker is programmed to stimulate the atria and then the ventricles in succession. The first spike depolarizes the atria, and after a brief interval, the _____ are stimulated by a separate ventricular stimulus.

ventricles

NOTE: Some modern pacemakers have physiological sensors which can detect, and respond to, the need for an increase in the rate of pacing. Other pacemakers now have the capability of detecting arrhythmias, and some can respond with a cardioversion stimulus or even defibrillate the ventricles as necessity dictates.

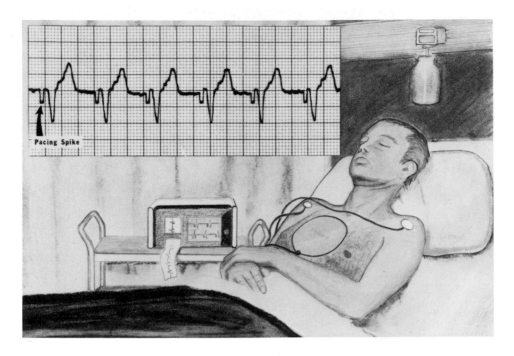

There are emergency pacemaking devices which can deliver stimuli to the heart through the intact skin of the chest.

Sophisticated pacemakers are available to painlessly pace the heart through intact _____. These *external non-invasive* pacemakers are ideal for emergency pacing needs.

skin

Pacing from the body surface requires an impulse of longer duration than that of intracardiac electrodes, so each pacing spike is wide with a _____ end.

flat

This makes possible immediate (emergency) pacemaking potential without surgical intervention, which can sustain many lives until a permanent pacemaker can be surgically _____.

implanted

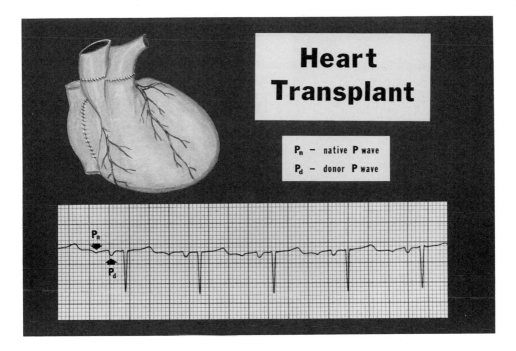

A heart transplant procedure leaves a portion of the original "native" upper atria in place, so a transplant patient will have his native SA Node and the transplant's SA Node.

NOTE: To be expeditious during these procedures, the portions of the native atria which are joined to large vessels are left behind to be sutured to the atria of the transplanted heart. Due to the position of the SA Node, it remains behind as well. Myocardial incisions insulate [electrically] the rejoined areas from one-another.

Transplant patients therefore have two SA Nodes producing independent _____ waves.

P

The "native" SA Node discharges are independent and usually not conducted to the transplanted _____.

heart

The transplanted heart has its own functional SA Node which controls the heart's pacing activity, so its P waves are followed by _____ complexes.

QRS

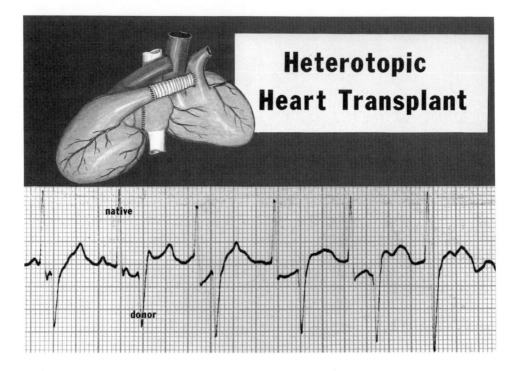

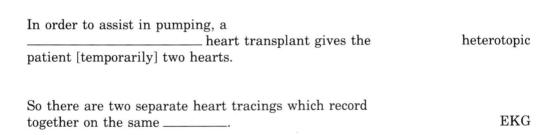

A *heterotopic* heart transplant is a procedure in which the native heart remains in place, and a temporary donor heart is surgically attached to assist the pumping effort.

In order to assist in pumping, a
_____ heart transplant gives the   heterotopic
patient [temporarily] two hearts.

So there are two separate heart tracings which record
together on the same _____.   EKG

> NOTE: To assist pumping, *artificial* [mechanical] implants
> are becoming more common as the sophistication of bio-
> engineering advances continue to improve. It is unlikely
> that a totally artificial heart will ever approach the
> efficacy and safety of that designed by Nature.

Cardiac Monitor Displays

Cardiac monitors display the same information as recorded on a standard 12 lead EKG. Some initial apprehension may arise because of lack of familiarity with the display. There is an increased amplitude of waves (height and depth) as well as a reversal of customary black tracing on white EKG paper, and some monitors lack a background grid. But don't dispair, this is just another method of displaying the heart's electrical activity . . . and familiarity eventually breeds *content*.

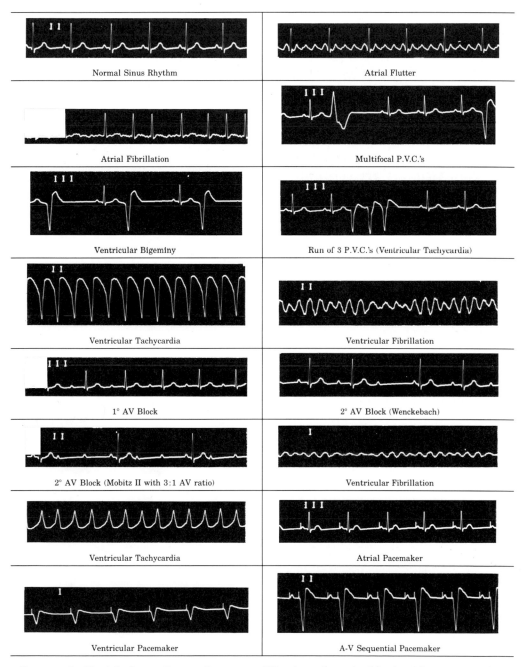

Normal Sinus Rhythm	Atrial Flutter
Atrial Fibrillation	Multifocal P.V.C.'s
Ventricular Bigeminy	Run of 3 P.V.C.'s (Ventricular Tachycardia)
Ventricular Tachycardia	Ventricular Fibrillation
1° AV Block	2° AV Block (Wenckebach)
2° AV Block (Mobitz II with 3:1 AV ratio)	Ventricular Fibrillation
Ventricular Tachycardia	Atrial Pacemaker
Ventricular Pacemaker	A-V Sequential Pacemaker

Because the "leads" of a cardiac monitor are modifications of standard leads with exaggerated amplitudes to aid in visualization at a distance, voltage (height and depth) criteria can not be utilized.

Monitor Displays Courtesy of:
Marquette Electronics, Inc.
Milwaukee, WI, U.S.A.

Electrocardiography was your challenge.

Knowledge is your achievement.

Now that you are certainly pleased with your understanding of basic electrocardiography, and proud of your new ability to interpret EKG's, you must realize how logical and marvelously designed is the heart.

You should be ready for *Rapid Comprehension of EKG's* for a more in-depth and comprehensive (yet simplified) approach to electrocardiography. Motivated?

Cover Publishing Co.
P.O. Box 1092
Tampa, FL 33601
U.S.A.

(pages 279 to 292)

from: Dubin's *Rapid Interpretation of EKG's*
published by: Cover Publishing Co., P.O. Box 1092, Tampa, FL 33601, USA

The owner of this book is encouraged to copy pages 279 through 292 to carry as a personal quick reference, however copying for or by others is strictly prohibited. The entire text of *Rapid Interpretation of EKG's* is fully protected by domestic United States copyright as well as the Universal Copyright Convention, and all rights of absolute imprimatur are enforced by COVER Publishing Co.

RAPID
INTERPRETATION
OF
EKG's

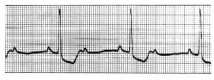

Dubin's classic, simplified methodology for understanding EKG's

Revised and **Updated**
4th Edition

Dale Dubin, M. D.

With the sophistication of modern copying machines, pages 279 to 292 may be reduced or enlarged to accommodate any personal-reference notebook with a minimum of redundancy in one dimension. Skillful copying of the front and back of each sheet can assure that the information is displayed effectively on both sides of seven sheets. Use a regular sheet of your notebook's paper to mark the holes once the sheets are copied.

May mankind benefit from your knowledge,

Dale Dubin

Dubin's Method
for
Reading EKG's

from: Dubin's *Rapid Interpretation of EKG's*
published by: Cover Publishing Co., P.O. Box 1092, Tampa, FL 33601, USA

1. RATE (pages 48–75)

Say "300,150,100" . . . "75,60,50"
- but for bradycardia:
  rate = Cycles/6 sec. strip × 10

2. RHYTHM (pages 76–157)

Identify the basic rhythm, then scan tracing for abnormal waves, pauses and irregularity.
- Check for P before each QRS
  "   QRS after each P
- Check P-R intervals (for AV Blocks)
  "   QRS interval (for B.B.B.)
- If Axis Deviation, rule out Hemiblock

3. AXIS (pages 158–196)

- QRS above or below baseline for Axis Quadrant (for Normal vs. R. or L. Axis Deviation).
- For Axis in degrees, find isoelectric QRS in a limb lead of Axis Quadrant.
- Axis rotation in the horizontal plane: (chest leads) find "transitional" (isoelectric) QRS.

4. HYPERTROPHY (pages 197–212)

Check V_1
- P wave for atrial hypertrophy
- R wave for R. Ventric. Hypert.
- S wave for L. Ventric. Hypert.
  . . . + R wave in V_5 for L.V.H.

5. INFARCTION (pages 213–256)

Scan all leads for:
- Q waves
- Inverted T waves
- ST segment elevation or depression

Find the location of the pathology (in the L. ventricle), and then identify the causative coronary artery.

Rate (pages 48 to 75)

from: Dubin's *Rapid Interpretation of EKG's*
published by: Cover Publishing Co., P.O. Box 1092, Tampa, FL 33601, USA

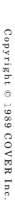

○ **Determine Rate by Observation** (pages 58 to 66)

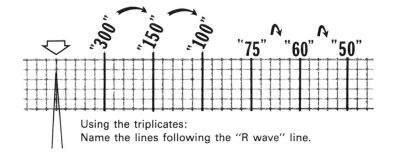

Using the triplicates:
Name the lines following the "R wave" line.

Fine division/Rate association: Reference (page 68)

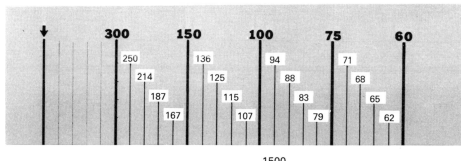

★ May be calculated: $\dfrac{1500}{\text{mm. between similar waves}}$ = RATE

Bradycardia (slow rates) (pages 69 to 75)

- Cycles/6 second strip × 10 = Rate
- When there are 10 large squares between similar waves, the rate is 30/minute.

Sinus Rhythm: origin is the SA Node ("Sinus Node"), normal rate 60 to 100/min.

- Rate more than 100/min. = *Sinus Tachycardia* (page 51)
- Rate less than 60/min. = *Sinus Bradycardia* (page 50)

Determine any co-existing, independent (atrial/ventricular) rates:

- Dissociated Rhythms: (pages 121, 143)
  A Sinus Rhythm can co-exist with an independent ectopic focal rhythm from another level. Determine rate of each.

Irregular Rhythms: (page 89)

- With Irregular Rhythms (such as Atrial Fibrillation) *always* note the general (average) ventricular rate (QRS's per 6-sec. strip times 10).

Rhythm (pages 76 to 157)

from: Dubin's *Rapid Interpretation of EKG's*
published by: Cover Publishing Co., P.O. Box 1092, Tampa, FL 33601, USA

★ **Identify basic rhythm . . .**

   . . . then scan entire tracing for abnormal waves, pauses, premature beats, and irregularity

★ **Always:**

- Check for P before each QRS
    "   "   QRS after each P
- Check PR intervals (for AV Blocks)
    "   QRS interval (for B.B.B.)
- Has QRS vector shifted outside normal range? (for Hemiblock)

Irregular Rhythms (pages 86 to 90)

Sinus Arrhythmia (page 87)

Irregular rhythm which varies with respiration.
All P waves are identical.
Considered normal.

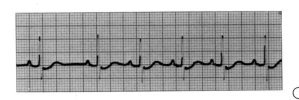

Wandering Pacemaker (page 88)

Irregular rhythm. P waves change shape as pacemaker location varies.

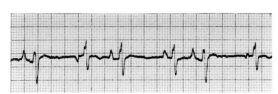

but if the rate exceeds 100/min, then it is called
Multifocal Atrial Tachycardia

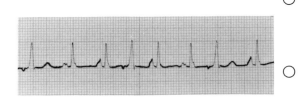

Atrial Fibrillation (pages 89, 130, 131)

Irregular ventricular rhythm.
Erratic atrial spikes (no P waves) from multiple atrial foci.
Atrial discharges may be difficult to see.

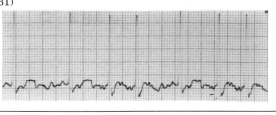

Rhythm cont. (pages 76 to 157)

from: Dubin's *Rapid Interpretation of EKG's*
published by: Cover Publishing Co., P.O. Box 1092, Tampa, FL 33601, USA

Escape—the heart's response to a pause in pacing (pages 91 to 100).

- An unhealthy Sinus (SA) Node may fail to emit a pacing stimulus; this "Sinus Block" results in a pause in a Sinus Rhythm.

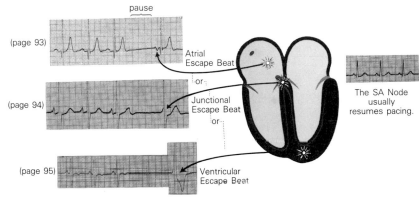

pause

(page 93) Atrial Escape Beat

or

(page 94) Junctional Escape Beat

or

(page 95) Ventricular Escape Beat

The SA Node usually resumes pacing.

- But a sick Sinus (SA) Node may cease pacing ("Sinus Arrest"), causing an ectopic focus to "escape" to assume pacemaker status.

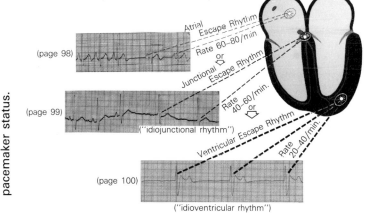

Atrial Escape Rhythm
Rate 60–80/min.

(page 98)

or

Junctional Escape Rhythm
Rate 40–60/min.

(page 99)

("idiojunctional rhythm")

or

Ventricular Escape Rhythm
Rate 20–40/min.

(page 100)

("idioventricular rhythm")

Premature Beats (pages 101 to 113)

- An ectopic focus may suddenly discharge producing a:

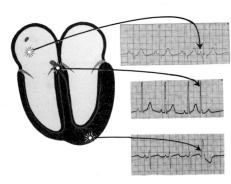

Premature Atrial Beat
(page 102)

Premature Junctional Beat
(page 103)

Premature Ventricular Contraction
(pages 104 to 112)
P.V.C.'s may be:
multiple, multifocal, in runs,
or coupled with normal cycles

Rhythm continued

from: Dubin's *Rapid Interpretation of EKG's*
published by: Cover Publishing Co., P.O. Box 1092, Tampa, FL 33601, USA

Rapid Ectopic Rhythms (pages 114 to 134)

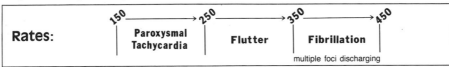

Rates: 150 → 250 → 350 → 450

Paroxysmal Tachycardia | Flutter | Fibrillation

multiple foci discharging

Paroxysmal (sudden) Tachycardia . . . rate: 150–250/min.
(pages 115 to 123)

"Supraventricular Tachycardia" (page 120)

Paroxysmal Atrial Tachycardia (page 117)

Atrial focus discharging at 150–250/min. producing normal wave sequence, when P′ waves are visible.

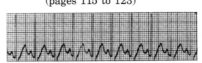

- ### P.A.T. with block (page 118)

  Same as P.A.T. but only every second (or more) P′ wave produces a QRS

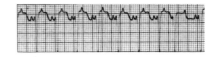

Paroxysmal Junctional Tachycardia

AV Junctional focus produces a rapid sequence of QRS-T cycles at 150–250/min. QRS may be slightly widened. (page 119)

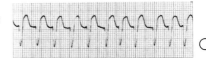

Paroxysmal Ventricular Tachycardia

(pages 121 to 123)
Ventricular focus produces a rapid (150–250/min) sequence of (P.V.C.-like) wide ventricular complexes.

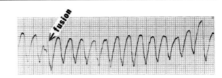

Flutter . . . rate: 250–350/min. (pages 124 to 127)

Atrial Flutter (pages 124, 125)

A continuous ("saw tooth") rapid sequence of atrial complexes from a single rapid-firing atrial focus. Many flutter waves needed to produce a ventricular response.

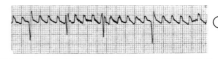

Ventricular Flutter (pages 126, 127)

A rapid series of smooth sine waves from a single rapid-firing ventricular focus; usually in a short burst leading to Ventricular Fibrillation.

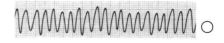

Fibrillation . . . erratic [multifocal] rapid discharges at 350 to 450/min. (pages 129 to 134)

Atrial Fibrillation (pages 130, 131)

Multiple atrial foci rapidly discharge producing a jagged baseline of tiny spikes. Ventricular (QRS) response is irregular.

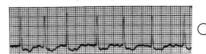

Ventricular Fibrillation (pages 132 to 134)

Multiple ventricular foci rapidly discharge producing a totally erratic ventricular rhythm without identifiable waves. Needs immediate treatment.

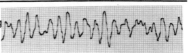

Rhythm continued

from: Dubin's *Rapid Interpretation of EKG's*
published by: Cover Publishing Co., P.O. Box 1092, Tampa, FL 33601, USA

("Heart") Blocks (pages 135 to 156)

Sinus (SA) Block (page 136) An unhealthy Sinus (SA) Node misses one or more cycles (sinus pause) . . .

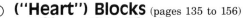

. . . the Sinus Node usually resumes pacing, but the pause may evoke an "escape" response from an ectopic focus (see page 283).

Always check:
- are P-R intervals less than one large square?
- is every P wave followed by a QRS?

AV Block (pages 137 to 144) blocks which delay or prevent atrial impulses from reaching the ventricles.

1° AV Block . . . prolonged P-R interval (pages 138, 139).
P-R interval is prolonged to greater than .2 sec (one large square).

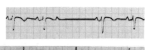

2° AV Block . . . some P's without QRS response (pages 140 to 142)

Wenckebach: P-R gradually increases with each
(page 140). cycle until the last P wave in the series does not produce a QRS.

Mobitz II: Some P's don't produce a QRS
(page 141) response. May appear like an occasional dropped QRS.

The same block may persist as a repeating 2:1 (AV) pattern (page 142).

More advanced block may produce a 3:1 (AV) pattern or even higher AV ratio (page 142).

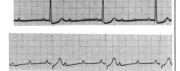

3° ("complete") AV Block . . . no P's produce a QRS response
(pages 143, 144)

3° Block: P waves—SA Node origin.
(page 144) QRS's—if narrow, then Junctional focus origin.

3° Block: P waves—SA Node origin.
(page 143) QRS's—if P.V.C.-like, then Ventricular focus origin.

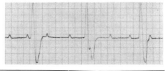

Bundle Branch Block . . . find R,R' in right or left chest leads
(pages 145 to 155)

Always Check:
- is QRS within 3 tiny squares?

QRS in Right B.B.B. (page 150)   QRS in Left B.B.B. (page 151)

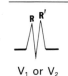

R R'

V₁ or V₂

With Bundle Branch Block the criteria for ventricular hypertrophy are unreliable

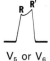

R R'

V₅ or V₆

Caution:
With Left B.B.B. infarction is difficult to determine.

"Hemiblock" . . . block of *Anterior* or *Posterior* fascicle of the Left Bundle Branch (pages 245 to 254).

Always Check:
- has Axis shifted outside Normal range?

Anterior Hemiblock (pages 247 to 249)   Posterior Hemiblock (pages 250, 251)

Axis shifts Leftward → L.A.D.   Axis shifts Rightward → R.A.D.
look for Q₁S₃   look for S₁Q₃

Axis (pages 158 to 196)

from: Dubin's *Rapid Interpretation of EKG's*
published by: Cover Publishing Co., P.O. Box 1092, Tampa, FL 33601, USA

General Determination of Electrical Axis (pages 158 to 185)
Is QRS positive (∧) or negative (∨) in leads I and AVF?

Is Axis Normal? (page 181)

QRS in lead I (pages 169 to 176)
. . . if QRS is Positive (mainly above baseline), then Vector points to positive (patient's left) side.

Lead I

Normal: { QRS upright in I and AVF / **"double thumbs-up sign"** }

QRS in lead AVF (pages 177–180)
. . . if the QRS is mainly Positive, then Vector must point downward to positive half of sphere.

Lead AVF

Determine Axis Quadrant
(pages 169 to 185)

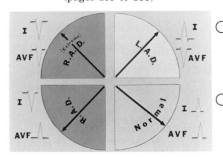

Axis in Degrees (pages 186 to 188)
After locating Axis Quadrant, find limb lead where QRS is most isoelectric:

Extreme Right Axis Deviation

lead	Axis
I →	−90°
AVL →	−120°
III →	−150°
AVF →	−180°

Right Axis Deviation

lead	Axis
AVF →	+180°
II →	+150°
AVR →	+120°
I →	+90°

Left Axis Deviation

lead	Axis
I →	−90°
AVR →	−60°
II →	−30°
AVF →	0°

Normal Range

lead	Axis
AVF →	0°
III →	+30°
AVL →	+60°
I →	+90°

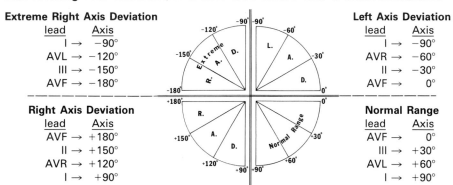

Axis Rotation (left/right) in the Horizontal Plane (pages 195, 196)
Find transitional (isoelectric) QRS in a chest lead.

transitional QRS
(isoelectric)

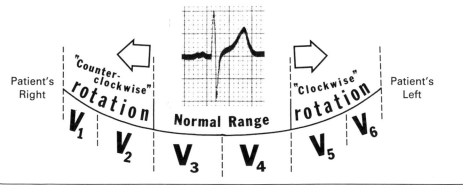

Patient's Right

"Counter-clockwise" rotation

V_1 V_2 V_3 **Normal Range** V_4

"Clockwise" rotation

Patient's Left

V_5 V_6

Hypertrophy (pages 197 to 212)

from: Dubin's *Rapid Interpretation of EKG's*
published by: Cover Publishing Co., P.O. Box 1092, Tampa, FL 33601, USA

Atrial Hypertrophy (pages 199 to 203)

Right Atrial Hypertrophy (page 202)

- large, diphasic P wave with tall initial component.

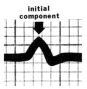

Left Atrial Hypertrophy (page 203)

- large, diphasic P wave with wide terminal component.

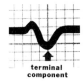

Ventricular Hypertrophy (pages 204 to 210)

Right Ventricular Hypertrophy (pages 204 to 206)

- R wave greater than S in V_1, but R wave gets progressively smaller from V_1–V_6.
- S wave persists in V_5 and V_6.
- R.A.D. with slightly widened QRS.

Left Ventricular Hypertrophy (pages 207 to 210)

$$\begin{array}{l} \text{S wave in } V_1 \text{ (in mm.)} \\ + \text{ R wave in } V_5 \text{ (in mm.)} \\ \hline \end{array}$$

   Sum in mm. is more than 35 mm. (for L.V.H.)

- L.A.D. with slightly widened QRS
- Inverted T wave:

slants downward slowly

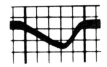

up rapidly

Infarction (pages 213 to 256)

from: Dubin's *Rapid Interpretation of EKG's*
published by: Cover Publishing Co., P.O. Box 1092, Tampa, FL 33601, USA

Q wave = Infarction (significant Q's only) (pages 225 to 228)

Q

- Significant Q wave is one millimeter (one small square) wide, which is .04 sec. in duration.
  —or is a Q wave $\frac{1}{3}$ the amplitude (or more) of the QRS complex.

- Note those leads (omit AVR) where significant Q's are present . . . see next page for determining infarct location, and identifying coronary vessel involved.

- Old infarcts: Q waves (like infarct damage) remain for a lifetime. To determine if an infarct is acute see below.

ST (segment) *Elevation* = (acute) Injury (pages 220 to 224) (also Depression)

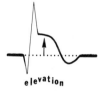
elevation

- Signifies an *acute* process, ST segment returns to baseline with time.

- ST Elevation associated with Q waves indicates an acute (or recent) infarct.

- A tiny "non-Q wave infarction" is noted as significant ST segment Elevation without associated Q's. Locate (next page) by identifying leads where it occurs.

- ST *Depression* (persistent) can represent "subendocardial infarction" which involves a small, shallow area just beneath the endocardium lining the left ventricle. This is also a variety of "non-Q wave infarction." Locate in the same manner (next page).

T wave Inversion = Ischemia (pages 218, 219)

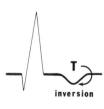
T
inversion

- Inverted T wave (of ischemia) is symmetrical (left half and right half are mirror images). Normally T wave is upright when QRS is upright.

- Usually associated in the same leads with acute (ST Elevation) infarction (Q waves)

- Isolated (non-infarction) ischemia may also be located by noting those leads where T wave inversion occurs, then identify which coronary vessel is narrowed.

★ Always obtain patient's previous EKG's for comparison!

Infarction Location
— and —
Coronary Vessel Involvement

(pages 241 to 256)

from: Dubin's *Rapid Interpretation of EKG's*
published by: Cover Publishing Co., P.O. Box 1092, Tampa, FL 33601, USA

Coronary Artery Distribution (page 241)

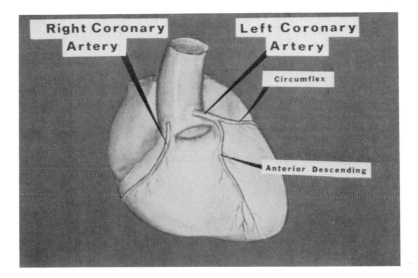

Infarction Location/Coronary Vessel Involvement (pages 241 to 256)

Posterior
- large R with
  ST Depression in V_1 & V_2
- mirror test
(Right Coronary Artery)
pages 234 to 238, 243.

Lateral
Q's in I and AVL
(Circumflex Coronary Artery)
pages 230, 242.

Inferior
(diaphragmatic)
Q's in II, III, and AVF
(R. or L. Coronary Artery)
pages 231, 244

Anterior
Q's in
V_1, V_2, V_3, and V_4
(Anterior Descending
  Coronary Artery)
pages 229, 242.

Miscellaneous (pages 257–276)

from: Dubin's *Rapid Interpretation of EKG's*
published by: Cover Publishing Co., P.O. Box 1092, Tampa, FL 33601, USA

Pulmonary Embolism (pages 259, 260)

- $S_1Q_3L_3$—wide S in I, and large Q and inverted T in III.
- acute Right B.B.B. (transient, often incomplete)
- R.A.D. and clockwise rotation
- Inverted T wave $V_1 \to V_4$ and ST depression in II

Artificial Pacemakers (pages 269 to 274)

Modern artificial pacemakers have sensing capabilities as well as provide a regular pacing stimulus. This electrical stimulus records on EKG as a tiny vertical spike which appears just before the "captured" cardiac response.

Demand Pacemakers: (page 272)

- are "triggered" (activated) when the patient's own rhythm ceases or slows markedly.

- are "inhibited" (cease pacing) if the patient's own rhythm resumes at a reasonable rate.

- will "reset" pacing (at same rate) to be synchronous with a premature beat.

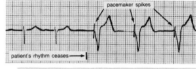

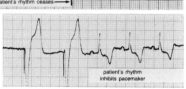

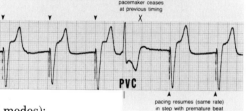

PVC

Pacemaker Impulse Delivery (variety of modes):

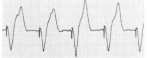

Ventricular Pacemaker (page 269)
(electrode in Right Ventricle)

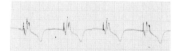

(Asynchronous) Epicardial Pacemaker (page 271)
Ventricular impulse *not* linked to atrial activity.

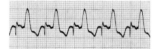

Atrial pacemaker (page 273)

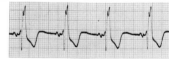

Atrial Synchronous Pacemaker (page 273)
P wave sensed, then after a brief delay,
ventricular impulse is delivered.

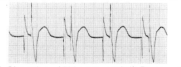

Dual Chamber (AV sequential) Pacemaker
(page 273)

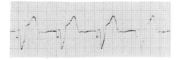

External Non-invasive Pacemaker (page 274)

Miscellaneous continued

from: Dubin's *Rapid Interpretation of EKG's*
published by: Cover Publishing Co., P.O. Box 1092, Tampa, FL 33601, USA

Electrolytes

Potassium (pages 261, 262)

- Increased K$^+$ (page 261)

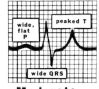

Moderate

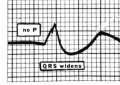

Extreme

- Decreased K$^+$ (page 262)

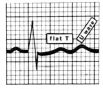

Moderate

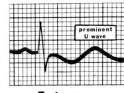

Extreme

Calcium (page 263)

Hyper Ca^{++}

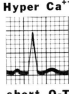

short Q-T

Hypo Ca^{++}

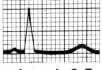

prolonged Q-T

Digitalis (pages 264 to 266)

- Appearance with digitalis (digitalis effect)
  Also:
  - T wave depressed or inverted.
  - Q-T interval shortened.

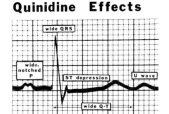

ST gradually slopes below baseline

- Digitalis Excess ⟶ Digitalis Toxicity
  (blocks)   (rapid ectopic discharge)
  - SA Block
  - P.A.T. with Block
  - AV Blocks
  - AV Dissociation
  - Atrial Fibrillation
  - Junctional or Ventricular Tachycardia
  - P.V.C.'s
  - Ventricular Fibrillation

Quinidine (pages 267, 268)

- Appearance with quinidine (page 267)

Quinidine Effects

wide QRS
wide, notched P
ST depression
U wave
wide Q-T

- Quinidine toxicity (page 268)

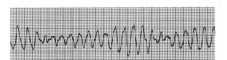

Torsades de Pointes

Practical Tips

from: Dubin's *Rapid Interpretation of EKG's*
published by: Cover Publishing Co., P.O. Box 1092, Tampa, FL 33601, USA

Dubin's Quickie Conversion
— for —
Patient's Weight in Pounds to Kilograms

Pt. wt. in kg. = Half of patient's wt. (in lb.) *minus* $\frac{1}{10}$ of that value.

Examples:	180 lb. pt. (becomes 90 *minus* 9) is 81 kg	160 lb. pt. (becomes 80 *minus* 8) is 72 kg	140 lb. pt. (becomes 70 *minus* 7) is 63 kg.

Modified Leads
— for —
Cardiac Monitoring

Locations are approximate. Some minor adjustment of electrode positions may be necessary to obtain the best tracing. Identify the specific lead on each strip placed in the patient's record.

		Identification	
Sensor Electrode		Letter	Color (inconsistent)
+		R (or RA)	white
−		L (or LA)	black
Ground (Neutral or Reference)		G (or RL)	variable

Modified Lead I

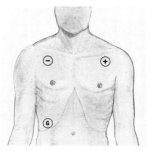

Modified Lead II

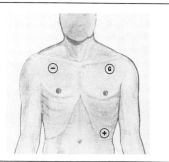

Conventional Lead

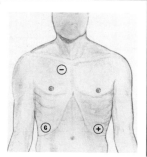

MCl₁
(To make this MCl₆ move ⊕ electrode to same (mirror) position on the patient's left side of the sternum)

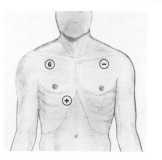

This section contains EKG tracings (and their interpretation) from various patients. The tracings and interpretations are provided so that you can see how this method of reading EKG's actually works. Try these few examples so that you will be accustomed to this systematic approach. Once you learn how to systematically read an EKG, you will soon become very skilled at routine EKG interpretations.

Patient D.D. is a 29 year old white male known to be a hypochondriac with numerous complaints.

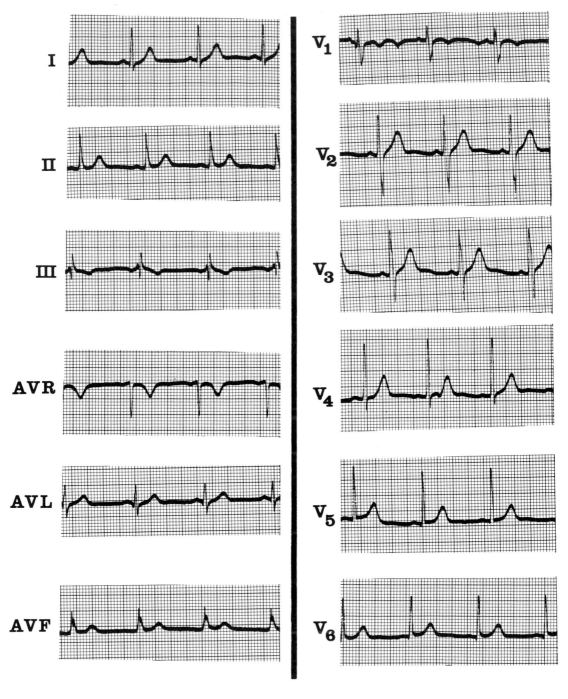

EKG Interpretation

Patient: D.D.

Rate: about 70 per minute

Rhythm: Regular Sinus Rhythm
    P-R less than .2 sec. (No AV Block)
    QRS less than .12 sec. (No B.B.B.)
        . . . but note the R,R′ in III suggesting incomplete Bundle Branch Block.

Axis: Normal Range (about +30°).
    Counter-clockwise rotation in the horizontal plane.

Hypertrophy: No atrial hypertrophy
        No ventricular hypertrophy

Infarction: No significant *Q waves*
  (coronary   *ST segments*—not elevated, except for V_5 and V_6 where ST is elevated
  vascular $^1/_2$mm. due to "early repolarization."*
  status)   *T waves*—generally upright

Comment: This is an essentially normal tracing. This is the author's own EKG, however he is no longer 29 years old.

*Early repolarization is characterized by (minimal) ST elevation in the left chest leads, often with counter-clockwise rotation (horizontal plane). It is a normal finding in young athletic males. This is covered in greater detail in *Rapid Comprehension of EKG's* (see page 278 in this book).

Patient R.C. is a 45 year old white male with a history of coronary vascular disease. Blood pressure was 210/100 on admission.

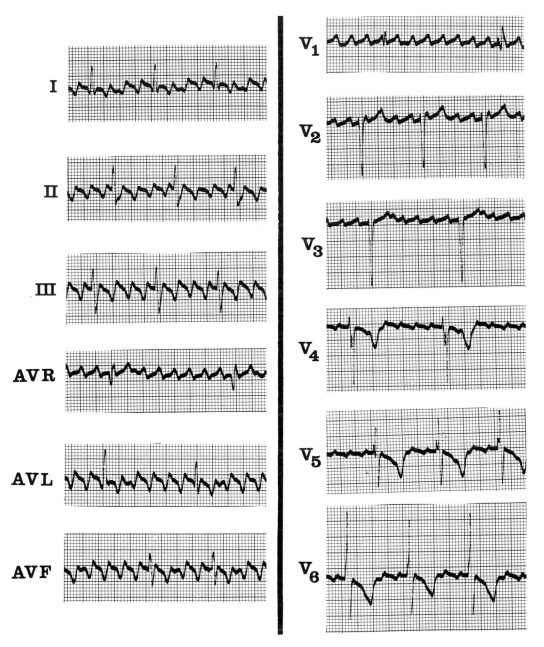

EKG Interpretation

Patient: R.C.

Rate: Atrial rate of 300/minute.
Ventricular rate generally 60/min. but occasionally slower.

Rhythm: Atrial Flutter (with inconsistent ventricular response, i.e. no fixed AV
ratio)
P-R is variable
QRS is less than .12 sec. (No B.B.B.)

Axis: Left Axis Deviation ($-30°$)
Clockwise rotation in the horizontal plane

Hypertrophy: Atrial hypertrophy difficult to determine.
No ventricular hypertrophy.

Infarction: *Q waves*—Q in lead I (also note large S in Lead III).
(coronary   *ST segments* are generally isoelectric.
vascular   *T waves* are inverted in I and AVL (look closely) and the mid-to-left
status)   chest leads.

Comment: The most obvious problem is Atrial Flutter with an atrial rate of 300/
min. and a variable irregular ventricular rate (average circa 60) caused
by the variable AV conduction ratio between 3:1 and 7:1. An old occlusion of the Left Circumflex Coronary artery is evidenced by the
old lateral infarction. New involvement of the Anterior Descending
Coronary artery is suggested by anterior ischemia (T wave inversion
in V_4, V_5, V_6), as well as by the probable Anterior Hemiblock (shift
to Left Axis Deviation with Q_1S_3 configuration; previously R.A.D. with
his old lateral M.I.). Note that if one scrutinizes the T wave regions
(somewhat obscured by flutter waves) in the limb leads, the flutter
waves dip lower (suggestive of negative T waves) rather than higher
(if superimposed on upright T waves) in all but AVR, indicating a
generalized cardiac ischemia, as well as the obvious compromise of
both branches of the Left coronary Artery.

Patient K.T. is a 61 year old obese male who was brought into the emergency room by his family. This patient had a sudden episode of severe left chest pain. Blood pressure was 95/65.

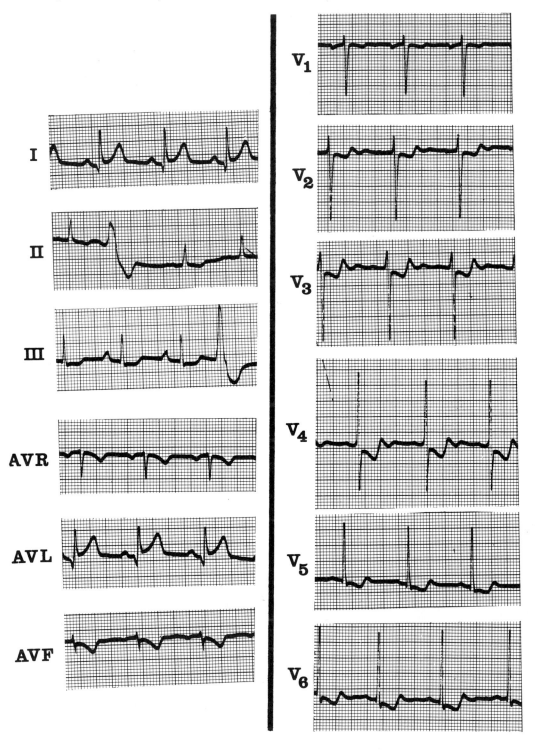

EKG Interpretation

Patient: K.T.

Rate: about 75/minute

Rhythm: Generally regular Sinus Rhythm with occasional P.V.C.'s.
  P-R is exactly .2 sec. so we will have to say there is a borderline first degree AV Block.
  QRS is less than .12 sec. (No B.B.B.).

Axis: Left Axis Deviation (nearly $-90°$).
  No rotation in the horizontal plane.

Hypertrophy: Probable left atrial hypertrophy.
  Left ventricular hypertrophy.

Infarction: *Significant Q waves* in I and AVL.
(coronary   *ST segments* are elevated in I and AVL. ST segments are depressed
vascular   in V_1, V_2, V_3, and V_4.
status)   *T waves* are flat or inverted in II, III, and AVF and all chest leads.

Comment: This patient has a classical acute lateral infarction caused by an occlusion of the Left Circumflex Coronary Artery. Coincident with this is a probable occlusion of the Right Coronary Artery characterized by prominent R waves with ST depression in the (V_1 to V_4) chest leads. Also T wave inversion in II, III and AVF suggests Right Coronary compromise. T wave inversion in all chest leads is indicative of ischemia of the Anterior Descending Coronary Artery. Note also the tall, peaked T waves in I and AVL known as "hyperacute T waves" which, although uncommon, are characteristic* of a very acute M.I. The Left Axis Deviation was seen in this patient's previous EKG's and is most likely related to his left ventricular hypertrophy rather than implicating Anterior Hemiblock (also, the Bundle Branch System appears to conduct normally). Occasional P.V.C.'s caused by the ischemia, depending on frequency and multiplicity of origin, may be foreboding of more serious arrhythmias.

*see *Rapid Comprehension of EKG's*

Patient G.G. is a 45 year old Black male who was doing heavy work when he was overcome by severe, crushing anterior chest pain. Blood pressure was 110/40 on admission to the hospital.

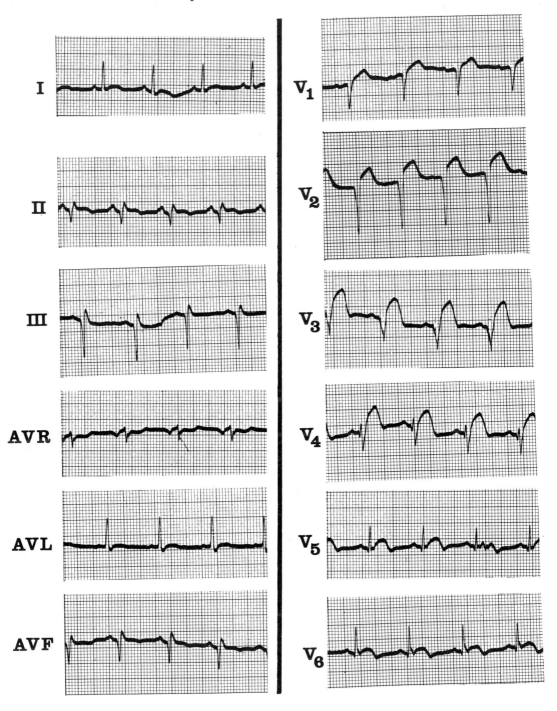

EKG Interpretation

Patient: G.G.

Rate: about 100/min. but variable.

Rhythm: Sinus Rhythm, somewhat irregular due to Sinus Arrhythmia.
        P-R less than .2 sec. (No AV Block)
        QRS less than .12 sec. (No B.B.B.)

Axis: Left Axis Deviation ($-30°$ to $-60°$).
      Clockwise rotation in the horizontal plane.

Hypertrophy: No atrial hypertrophy.
           No ventricular hypertrophy.

Infarction: *Significant Q waves* in II, III, and AVF.
(coronary   There are also very large Q waves in V_1, V_2, V_3, and V_4.
vascular   *ST segments* are elevated in V_1, V_2, V_3, and V_4.
status)   *T waves* are difficult to distinguish, but inverted T waves are noted
        in V_4, V_5, and V_6.

Comment: This patient has an acute antero-septal infarction probably representing an occlusion of the Anterior Descending branch of the Left
Coronary. Generalized ischemia of the myocardium is evident by the
flat-to-inverted T waves in nearly every lead. The old inferior infarction demonstrated on this EKG was noted on the patient's previous
hospital record and is the documented etiology of his Left Axis Deviation (no Hemiblock). Note that the QRS becomes isoelectric between V_4 and V_5 but this is *not* within the normal (V_3, V_4) range; this
represents minimal clockwise rotation away from the septal infarction. Old EKG's showed no anterior involvement on his previous
admission.

Patient E.M. is a 65 year old white female. She was admitted to the hospital because of constant left chest pain for twelve hours. Blood pressure on admission was 110/75.

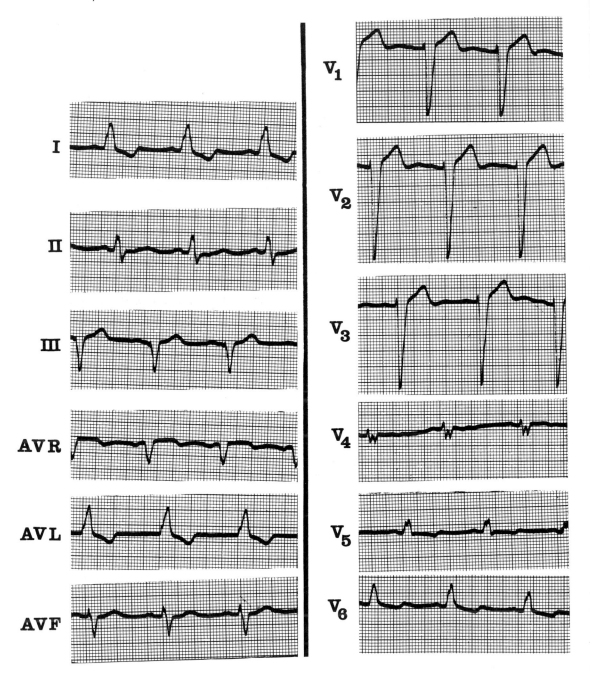

EKG Interpretation

Patient: E.M.

Rate: 60

Rhythm: Sinus Bradycardia
    $P\text{-}R$ is about .2 sec. and therefore there is probably a first degree AV
        Block.
    QRS is more than .12 sec. (it is .16 sec. wide). R,R' is present in V_5 and
        V_6 so there is a Left Bundle Branch Block.

Axis: Suggestive of Left Axis Deviation, but not reliable because of the presence
    of Bundle Branch Block.

Hypertrophy: No atrial hypertrophy
    Ventricular hypertrophy is difficult to determine because of Bun-
        dle Branch Block.

Infarction: *Q Waves*—not a reliable criterion of infarction in the presence of Left
(coronary   Bundle Branch Block.
vascular   *ST segments*—not reliable in the presence of Left Bundle Branch Block.
status)   *T Waves* are flat in V_4, V_5, and V_6, but not reliable with Left Bundle
        Branch Block.

Comment: Vectorcardiogram and enzyme studies confirmed a presumptive di-
    agnosis of myocardial infarction. A careful study of the patient's chest
    pains made us suspicious.

Patient M.A. is a 75 year old white female with a long history of marked hypertension.

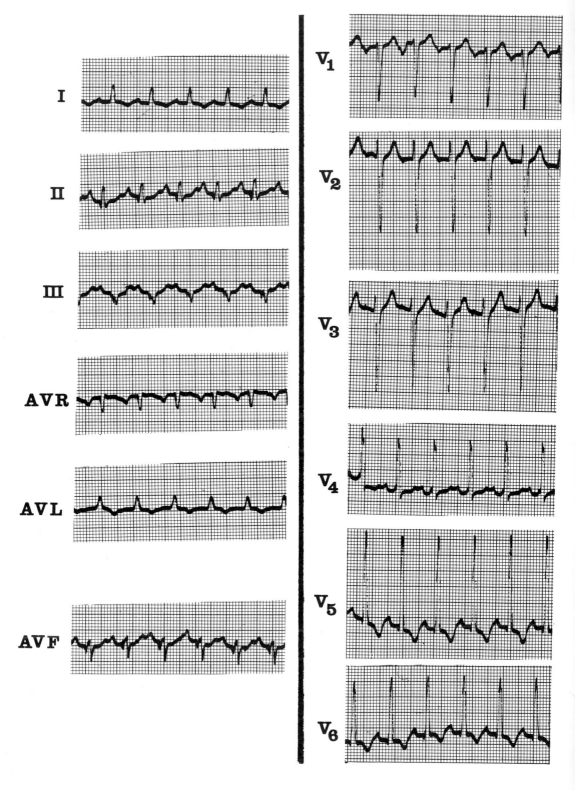

EKG Interpretation

Patient: M.A.

Rate: about 125/minute

Rhythm: Sinus Tachycardia
        P-R is less than .2 sec. (No AV Block)
        QRS is less than .12 sec. (No B.B.B.)

Axis: Left Axis Deviation (minimal amplitude of QRS in limb leads makes exact
      axis determination difficult).
      No rotation in the horizontal plane.

Hypertrophy: Left atrial hypertrophy
             Left ventricular hypertrophy with strain

Infarction: *Q waves* are present in II, III, and AVF.
(coronary   *ST segments*—generally isoelectric (on baseline), but V_5 and V_6 show
vascular   "strain" pattern.
status)   *T waves* are inverted in I and AVL, and also in V_5, V_6.

Comment: This patient has hypertrophy of both the left atrium and left ventricle
         with a left ventricular strain pattern. The patient also had an old
         inferior infarction. The Left Axis Deviation is caused by the Mean
         QRS Vector pointing away from the (old) inferior M.I. and toward the
         thickened left ventricle. It does *not* represent Hemiblock. There is cur-
         rently (lateral) ischemia in the distribution of the Left Circumflex
         Coronary Artery.

R.M., an anxious, obese 47 year old white male in a plastic surgeon's waiting room, complained of "tight, squeezing" pain in his anterior chest. An electrocardiogram was quickly taken with a portable EKG machine.

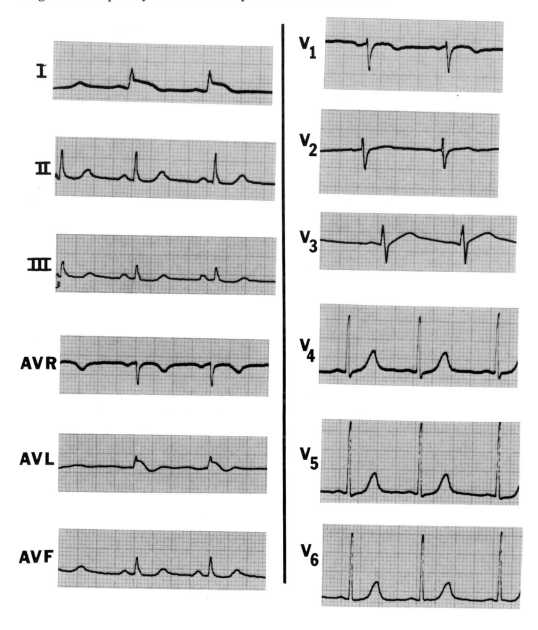

EKG Interpretation

Patient: R.M.

Rate: 75

Rhythm: Sinus Rhythm
  P-R .16 sec. (No AV Block)
  QRS .08 sec. (No B.B.B.)

Axis: about +45° (Normal)
  No rotation in the horizontal plane

Hypertrophy: Possible minimal left atrial hypertrophy
  No ventricular hypertrophy

Infarction: *Q waves*—no significant Q waves
  (coronary *ST segments*—elevated 2+ mm. in I and AVL
  vascular *T waves*—inverted in I and AVL.
  status)

Comment: It is interesting that in this innocuous appearing EKG there is a sub-
tle non-Q wave infarction in the lateral left ventricle which very soon
developed into a serious lateral infarction. The symptomatology
suggestive of M.I. always must be investigated and scrutinized.

Index